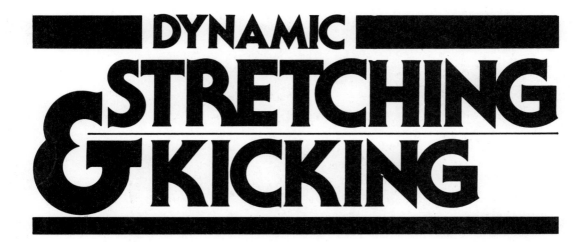

By BILL "SUPERFOOT" WALLACE

**U!P UNIQUE
PUBLICATIONS**

© **UNIQUE PUBLICATIONS, INC., 1982**
All rights reserved
Printed in the United States of America

ISBN: 0-86568-018-3
Library of Congress No.: 81-51824

DISCLAIMER

Contents

Introduction

"Dynamic Stretching and Kicking" is structured into two complete sections. The first section deals with stretching and agility as the key element for developing skill, strength and health. The second section deals exclusively with my kicking technique and strategy of sparring. Each of my three most famous kicks are analyzed in great detail and with their proper application. Stretching and kicking being the two most important aspects of my repertoire of skills, I sincerely hope that they will make a significant contribution to your own training and knowledge in the martial arts.

As odd as it may sound, please do not read this book. Rather, study it and live with it. I will have accomplished my purpose in writing this book, if it becomes for you a source of inspiration as well as a source of knowledge and skill.

Good luck in your training!

Bill Wallace

STRETCHING

Anatomy, Physiology, and Kinesiology of Flexibility

A muscle is made up of thousands of muscle fibers. These fibers are connected in bundles to form the body of the muscle. Muscles are then attached to the bones by tendons and ligaments. During a muscle contraction, one bone moves freely, while one bone remains stationary. The muscle attachment to the stationary bone, which will be closer to the midpoint of the body, is called the muscle's origin. The muscle attachment to the moveable bone, which will be further from the midpoint of the body, is called the insertion. The origin of the bicep muscle, for example, is the shoulder, and the insertion is the elbow.

Each muscle is either an adductor or an abductor. Adductor muscles bring the body back to normal alignment; abductor muscles pull the bones away from the body. For example, the quadriceps, which pulls the leg out, is an abductor muscle; the sartorius, which pulls the leg back in, is an adductor muscle. Note that the muscles always pull a bone—they never push.

When any movement occurs, the muscles which caused the movement work in pairs. One muscle acts as an agonist, while an opposing muscle acts as an antagonist. The agonist pulls the muscle to make the

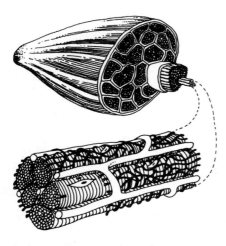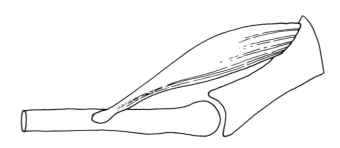

necessary movement. The antagonist muscle must relax and stretch; otherwise it works against the agonist. For example, when you bring your hand to your shoulder, the biceps do the work, and is thus the agonist. The antagonist is the triceps. If the triceps are tight, it's hard to pull the arm up. The same thing happens in splits. When performing this exercise, the agonist is the quadriceps, and the satorius (groin muscle) is the antagonist.

The joints are points where two or more bones meet and are covered by ligaments and tendons. If these attachments are overstretched, they will not shorten again like muscles, but will cause a permanent weakening of the joint. When exercising, it's important not to work against or overextend a joint.

The muscles are warmed and nourished by the blood supply pumped through the body. The blood also provides the muscles with oxygen and carries away lactic acid. Lactic acid is a waste product that accumulates in the muscles and makes them tired. When a muscle is tight, it will restrict the passage of blood through the capillaries and blood vessels. This means that a tight muscle will be getting much less blood circulation than a relaxed, flexible muscle. In a flexible person, the blood moves freely and the muscle can quickly get rid of its lactic acid buildup. It can also repair strains or bruises more quickly.

Major Muscle Groups

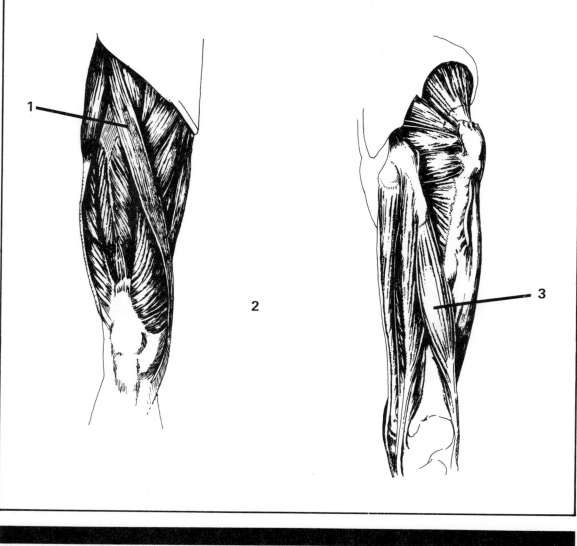

1. Sartorius
A narrow strap muscle which is the longest muscle in the body. Its insertion is the spine; its origin is the tibia. It assists in flexing the leg and it moves and rotates the thigh.

2. Quadriceps
This major extensor muscle of the leg consists of four parts. Its insertion is the fibula and tibia; its origin is the upper hip. This muscle is used to straighten the leg out and extend the leg from the thigh. When this muscle is the agonist, the biceps femoris is the antagonist.

3. Biceps Femoris
This muscle group is at the back of the upper leg. Its insertion is the fibular and tibia; its origin is the hip. It is used in flexing the lower leg; drawing the trunk upright from a stooping position and rotating the knee.

4. Gastrocnemius
This muscle is the "belly" of the calf. Its insertion is the ankle bone; its origin is the femur. It is used to rotate the foot and to propel the body forward in walking, running, and leaping.

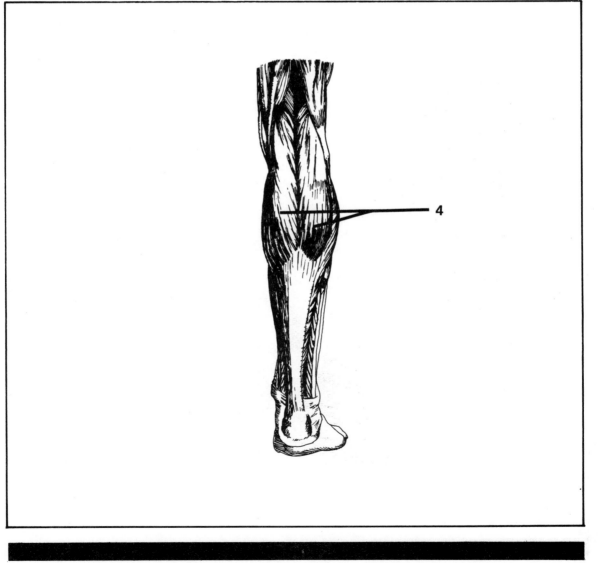

5. Trapezius

This muscle group extends over the back of the neck and upper back. Its insertion is the clavicle/scapula; its origin is the occipital bone. It is used to turn the head and work the shoulders.

6. Latissimus Dorsi

This is the major muscle of the upper body. Its insertion is the humerus; its origin is the vertebrae. It is used to lower, raise, and rotate the arms, and to depress the raised arm against resistance.

7. Lumbar Muscles

These are the muscles of the lower back. The insertion is the angles of the ribs; the origin is the vertebrae. These muscles keep the lower back erect and turn it from side to side.

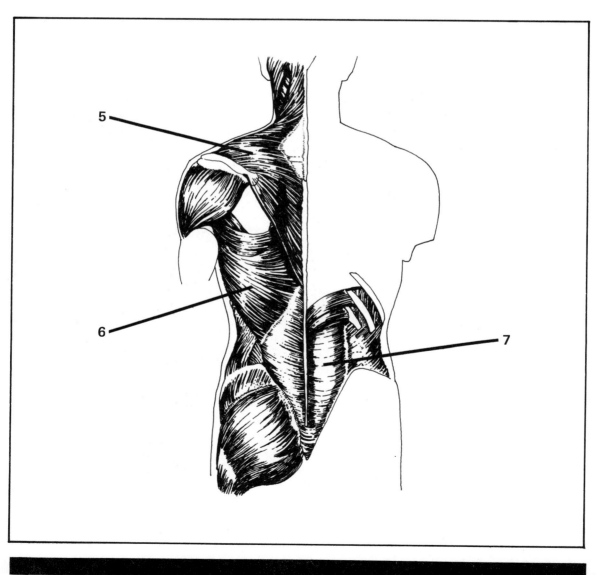

8. Pectoralis Major and Minor

These are the muscles of the chest. The insertion is the humerus; the origin is the sternum. These muscles are used to draw the arms forward and together, and are also used in climbing.

9. Deltoid

This is the shoulder muscle. Its insertion is the humerus; its origin is the clavicle/scapula. This muscle raises the arm to the side and draws the arm forward and backwards.

10. Biceps

This is the muscle of the upper arm. Its insertion is the radius and ulna; its origin is the clavicle/scapula. This muscle bends the arm and flexes the elbow joint.

11. Triceps

This is the arm extensor. Its insertion is the radius and ulna; its origin is the clavicle/scapula. This muscle straightens the arms, extends the forearm at the elbow joint, and is used in forward thrusting and pushing.

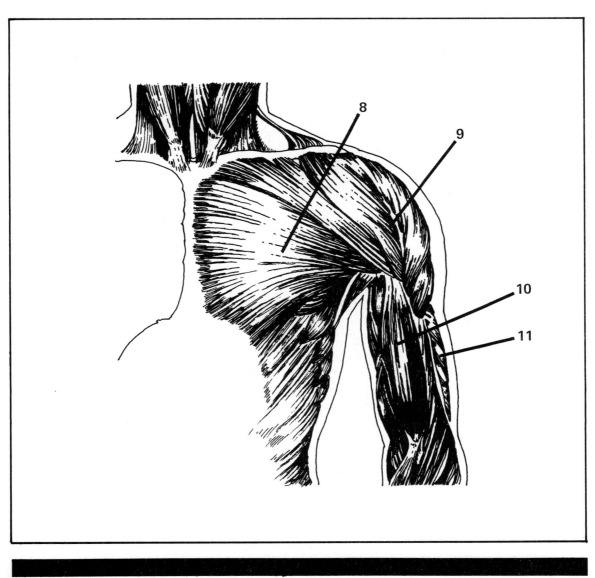

12. Forearm

The insertion is the eight bones in the wrist; the origin is the humerus. It is used for gripping and for moving the fingers and wrist.

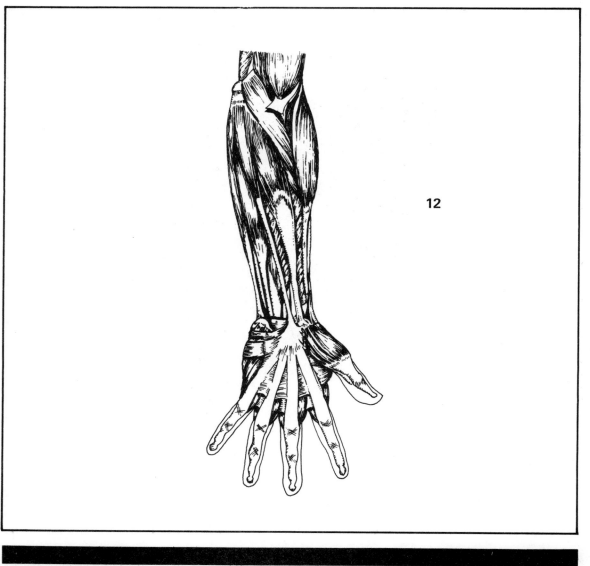

12

13. Abdominal Muscles

These are four large flat muscular sheets over the abdomen. The insertion and origin are the sternum, scapula, calvicle, and spine. This muscle keeps the internal organs in position. It is also used to bend the trunk forward and to draw the pelvis upwards.

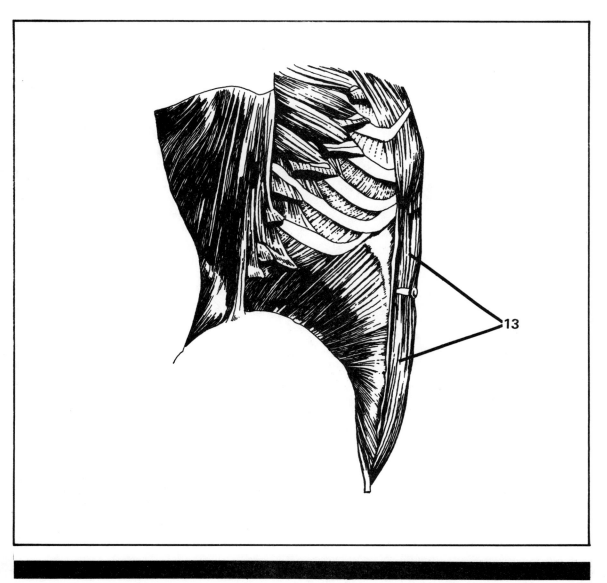

13

14. Neck

The insertion is the spine and vertebrae. The origin is the clavicle. This muscle turns the neck, and tilts and rotates the head.

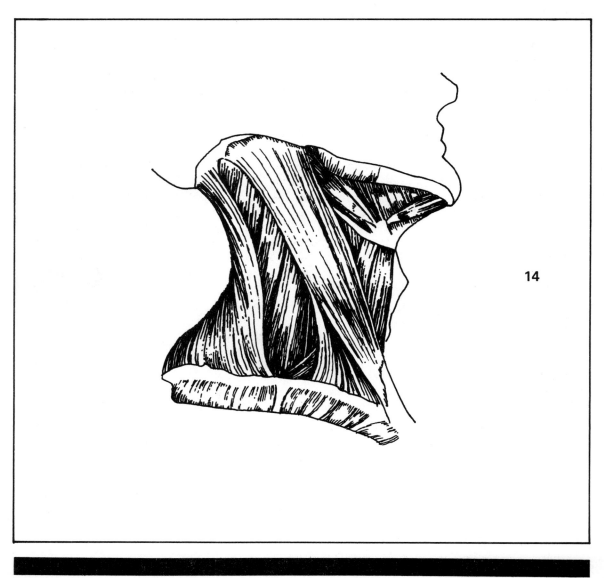

14

Benefits of Flexibility

Increased flexibility has been found essential in helping an athlete avoid injury, fatigue less quickly, and generally perform better.

When a person is flexible, each movement takes less work. The agonist, which does the work in any movement, does not have to exert as much force against the antagonist, since this muscle is looser and more relaxed. The athlete's energy can be focused on moving the agonist, thus generating more power in each movement.

Since the antagonist creates less resistance to movement, the agonist is able to contract more quickly. This enhances the athlete's speed.

Flexibility also helps prevent injuries. Most athletes are susceptible to muscle pulls, strains, and tears. Pulled hamstrings are particularly common. When muscles are tight, any quick movement or a movement beyond the normal range of the muscle will cause a strain or tear. A flexible athlete, however, will have relaxed muscles which can receive strains or hits without sustaining injuries.

Stamina will also be increased. Not only does the flexible athlete not have to work as hard, but because of an increased blood supply, more oxygen will be available to the muscles. The lactic acid, which accumulates in the muscles and makes them tired, will also be carried away faster. Distance runners, for example, need to have loose muscles for endurance, while sprinters may have tighter muscles, since they must release all of their energy in a short period of time.

How to Stretch

1. Never bend your back when you stretch. Always bend at the hips, keeping your lower back as straight as possible. The muscles in the lower back are particularly susceptible to tears. Unlike the strong, bulky muscles in the biceps, the lower back muscles are in thin sheets, which are hooked into the vertebrae. These sheets of muscles tear very easily, and may pull discs in the lower back out of position and push on nerves. This can cause debilitating pain in the lower back and lumbar region.

2. Don't work quickly. Remember that gaining flexibility takes time. Let your slow motions gently loosen the body and let the increased blood supply from stretching and relaxing work with you.

3. Remember not to bounce. Concentrate on exercising slowly and smoothly.

4. Work your muscles until you feel the tension. If you don't feel anything in your muscles, the exercise isn't doing anything for you. If you are so flexible already that you don't feel any tension in the beginning exercises, change the movement or your stance until you do feel tension. You may wish to hold a position for longer (up to 30 seconds); take a wider stance; or use weights or your own body weight to intensify the stretch.

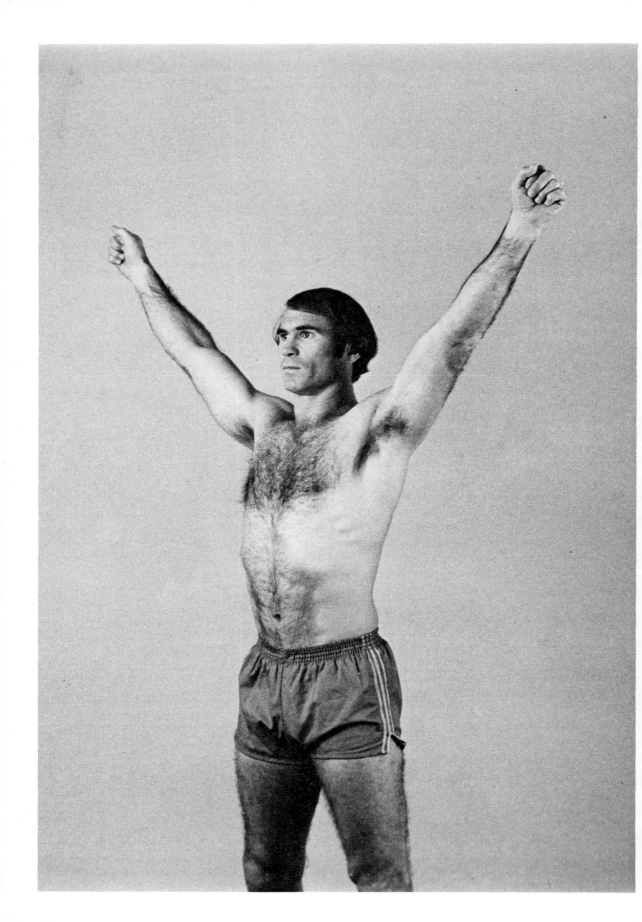

Warm Up Exercises

You must thoroughly warm up your body before embarking on any serious stretching exercises. This series of exercises systematically loosens and gently stretches all of the important muscle groups in your body. By spending fifteen to twenty minutes on these warm ups, your body will be prepared for the more demanding stretching exercises which follow, and you will be able to exert more pressure on muscles, tendons, and ligaments without causing injuries.

Neck Warm Up

The neck warm up is an excellent basic limbering exercise for the upper spine.

Number of Repetitions

5 to 10

Physiological Benefits

This exercise loosens all of the neck and shoulder muscles, and helps you eliminate tension in the shoulders. When done correctly, the exercise will help release the compression of the vertebrae and increase circulation to the brain.

Martial Arts Benefits

Relaxed shoulder muscles are essential for delivering powerful punches. Loose neck muscles help you evade or roll with punches or kicks to the head.

Pointers

Do not turn your head too quickly or vigorously when practicing this exercise. It is easy to pull a muscle or pinch a nerve in the back of your neck if this exercise is done carelessly. Develop the full range of motion in the neck.

Neck Warm Up

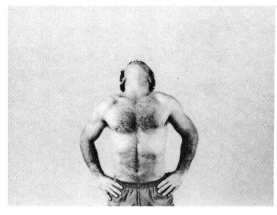

1. Move your head all the way back.

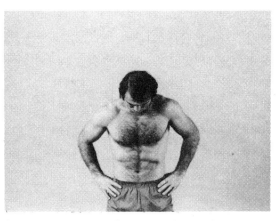

2. Move your head all the way forward . . .

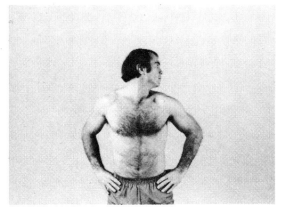

3. To the left . . .

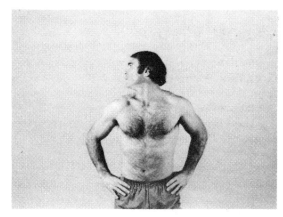

4. And all the way to the right.

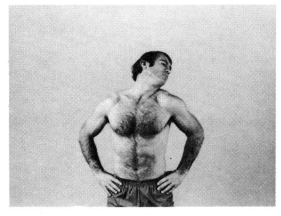

5. Roll you head to the left shoulder.

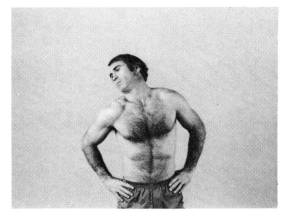

6. Roll your head to the right shoulder.

Shoulder Warm Up
Arm Circles

When loosening and strengthening the shoulder area, you should be aware that the shoulder includes not only the joint but the entire muscle complex, which extends into the upper arm, back, and neck. This exercise focuses on loosening the shoulder joint.

Number of Repetitions
10 repetitions for each size circle.

Physiological Benefits
This exercise helps you gain the maximum range of motion in your shoulder joint. The loosening effect also helps prevent nerves from being pinched in the ball and socket area. Your deltoid, pectorals, and trapezoid muscles will also be somewhat loosened and warmed up.

Martial Arts Benefits
Your arms must be loose in order to execute jabs, punches, and back fists quickly and powerfully. This exercise will also help improve your weaving motions, as your shoulders will easily move with your body.

Pointers
Be sure to practice this exercise very smoothly. You do not want to jerk or wrench the shoulder joint. Try not to use too much body movement, but make the shoulders do the work. Do not tense the shoulders but keep them relaxed throughout the entire exercise.

Shoulder Warm Up—Arm Circles

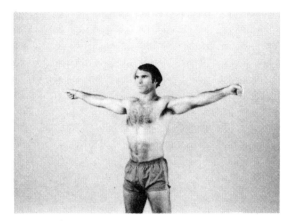

1. Stretch your arms straight out.

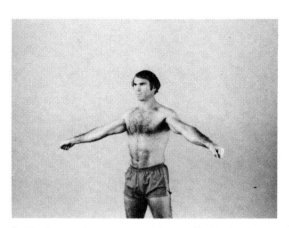

2. Begin moving your arms in small, clockwise circles.

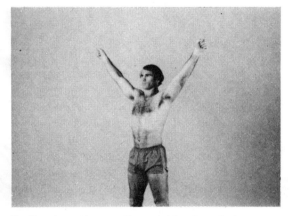

3. Continue the rotation, making ten circles.

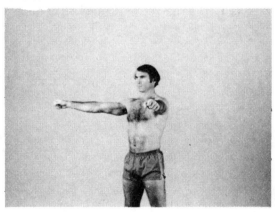

4. Begin to move your arms in slightly larger circles.

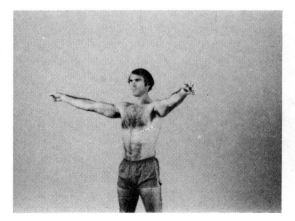

5. Make ten of these circles.

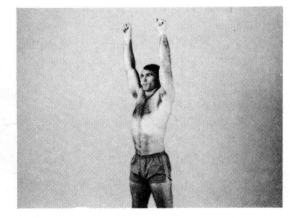

6. Now begin to move your arms in the largest circles possible.

Shoulder Warm Up
Arm Cross

This exercise concentrates on loosening all of the muscles in the shoulders, upper back, and chest area. Stiff shoulders can have a negative effect on your entire body, leading to stiff joints and bad posture.

Number of Repetitions

5-10

Physiological Benefits

The muscles of the chest will be expanded and the sternum itself will be loosened when this exercise is practiced correctly. You will also loosen the upper back muscles and gently stretch the spinal column.

Martial Arts Benefits

By relaxing your shoulder and upper body muscles, your fighting posture will be improved. Looseness of the upper body is vital for blocking, weaving, and executing quick jabs.

Pointers

Use a slow, steady movement when performing this exercise; never snap your arms. You can easily pull a chest or back muscle if the exercise is done incorrectly. The shoulders should be relaxed, keeping the breathing calm and regular.

Shoulder Warm Up—Arm Cross

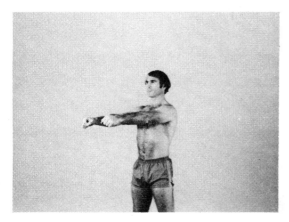

1. Hold your arms straight out in front of you.

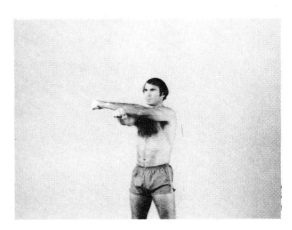

2. Swing your arms to cross them in front of you.

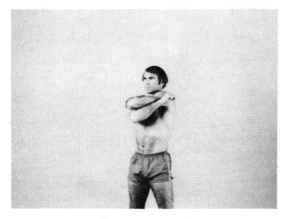

3. Continue the crossing motion to the point of tension.

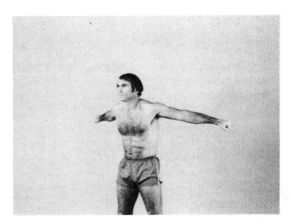

4. Return your arms to the original position.

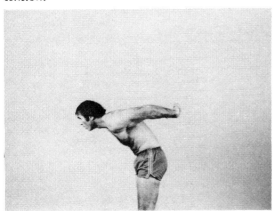

5. Now cross your arms behind you until the touch.

Elbow Warm Up #1

The elbow must be put through its full range of motion or the strength and flexibility of the arm will be affected. Exercises such as this one help lubricate the joint and keep the arm flexible.

Number of Repetitions

5-10

Physiological Benefits

In addition to keeping the biceps, triceps, and forearm muscles stretched and the joint functioning freely, this exercise helps improve circulation in the arms.

Martial Arts Benefits

This exercise prepares the arm for punching, blocking or any technique requiring fast arm movements.

Pointers

Never snap or hyperextend the elbow joint. It is important to keep the shoulders relaxed and level. The breathing should be quiet and calm. Tensing and raising the shoulders or improper breathing will cause unnecessary pressure against the elbows in the execution of this exercise.

Elbow Warm Up #1

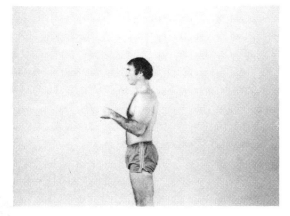

1. Bend your arms at the elbow.

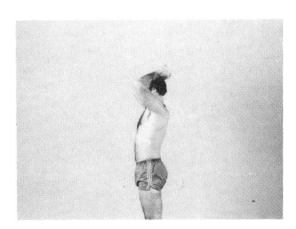

2. Keeping your elbows bent, bring your arms over your head.

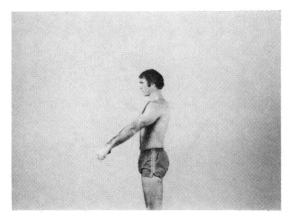

3. Bring your arms down, extending your arms with the downward movement.

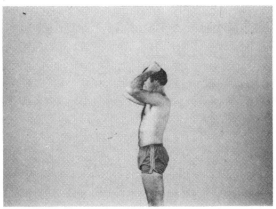

4. Repeat the exercise. Do not snap your arms in the extension.

Elbow Warm Up #2

Number of Repetitions
10-15
Physiological Benefits
This exercise is particularly good for breaking up any calcium deposits which may restrict arm movements.
Martial Arts Benefits
With an increased range of motion in the elbow joint, you will find it easier to move quickly from technique to technique, as from a jab to a backfist to a ridge hand or from a block to an attack.
Pointers
Do not grab the elbow joint during the exercise; it should only be supported by your other arm.

Elbow Warm Up #2

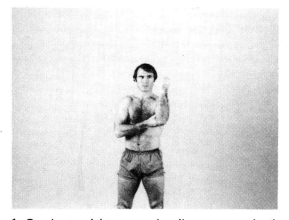

1. Bend your right arm at the elbow, supporting it with the other arm.

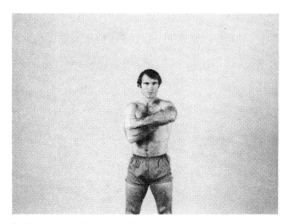

2. Begin moving your forearm in a counterclockwise circle.

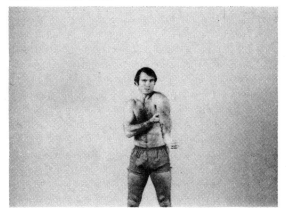

3. Bend it around . . .

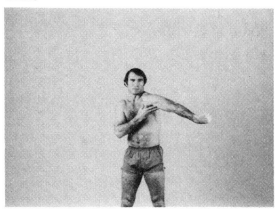

4. And back.

Wrist Warm Up #1

It is obvious that no hand technique can be executed effectively unless the wrist joint is properly lubricated and flexible.

Number of Repetitions

10

Physiological Benefits

By loosening the wrist joint, this exercise helps loosen the entire hand. This flexibility helps prevent damage or strain to the hand's tendons and nerves.

Martial Arts Benefits

This exercise is excellent in preparing for combinations, as when you smoothly move from open hand techniques such as a knife hand, ridge hand, or a slap, to closed hand techniques, such as punches, jabs, and backfists.

Pointers

Do not hold the wrist joint tightly, but concentrate on relaxing the joint and hand. It is important to concentrate on developing the full range of movement of the wrist.

Wrist Warm Up #1

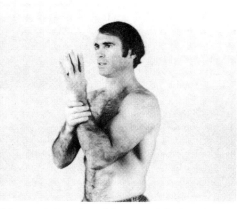

1. Hold your left wrist with your right hand.

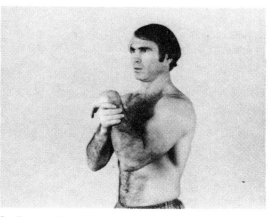

2. Rotate the hand down . . .

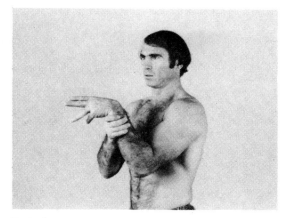

3. Left . . .

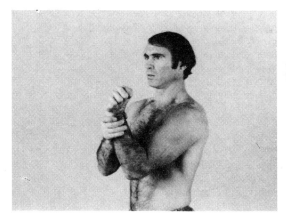

4. And back.

Finger Warm Up #1

Most exercise programs ignore the importance of finger joints. However, they must also be lubricated and moved through their full range of motion in order to improve gripping or manipulating techniques.

Number of Repetitions

10 (5 in each direction)

Physiological Benefits

By practicing this exercise whenever you have a free moment, you will loosen and strengthen the entire hand, including the wrist joint, finger joints, and tendons and muscles of the hand. This exercise also stretches the muscles of the forearm.

Martial Arts Benefits

You should find that grabs, foreknuckle strikes and other finger strikes are improved.

Pointers

Do not try to overextend the fingers in practicing this exercise.

Finger Warm Up #1

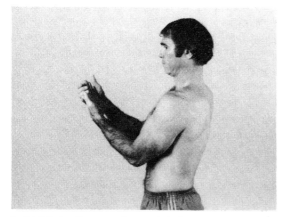

1. Hold the fingers of your left hand in your right hand.

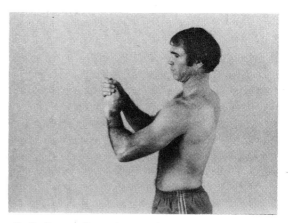

2. Pull your fingers towards your body.

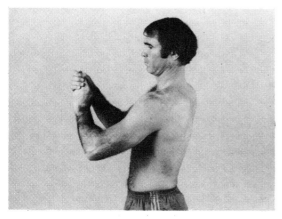

3. Pull your fingers away from your body.

Finger Warm Up #2

This exercise can be practiced anytime, and is particularly excellent when done with a slow, steady pressure which strains muscle against muscle.

Number of Repetitions
10

Physiological Benefits
Not only are the fingers, hands, wrist, and forearms strengthened, but the biceps, triceps, deltoids and chest muscles will also be developed when the exercise is practiced correctly.

Martial Arts Benefits
Grabs, strikes, and blocks will be improved.

Pointers
Do not allow your fingers or hands to cramp by exerting too much pressure.

Finger Warm Up #2

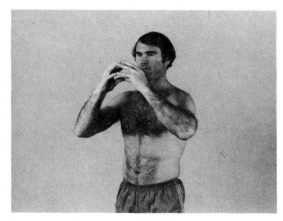

1. Put your fingers together, forming an arch.

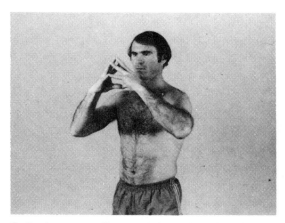

2. Push on your fingers to the point of tension. Hold.

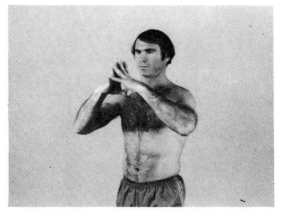

3. Slowly flatten the fingers, maintaining the tension.

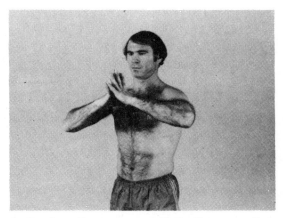

4. Continue the pressure until the fingers are flat against each other.

Finger Warm Up #3

As you practice these finger exercises, you will find that all of your hand techniques become more powerful.

Number of Repetitions
10

Physiological Benefits
This exercise strengthens the muscles and tendons of the hands and forearms.

Martial Arts Benefits
Note how your grabs improve as your forearms and hands become more powerful.

Finger Warm Up #3

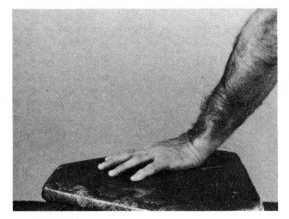 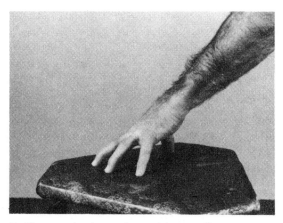

1. Put your hand flush against a flat surface.

2. Try to grip the surface with your fingers.

Hip Warm Up #1

As noted earlier, the hip is the largest joint in the body, and one of the most important. It is your center of balance, and the central hinge between the upper torso and the legs. All leg and upper body movement are dependent on flexibility in the hips.

Number of Repetitions

10-15

Physiological Benefits

As the hip joint is moved through its full range of motion, you will release compression in the lower spinal column and loosen the muscles of the lower back, abdominals, and oblique muscles.

Martial Arts Benefits

This exercise is particularly valuable in bringing the knee up and holding it high and close to the body in preparation for a kick. Loose hips also help improve all aspects of footwork, including maneuvering, turning, dodging, and evading.

Pointers

Be careful to avoid putting too much pressure on the knees, as it is easy to strain the joint and outer knee muscles. Practice the exercise at a moderate speed, but make sure you are still concentrating on developing the full range of motion.

Hip Warm Up #1

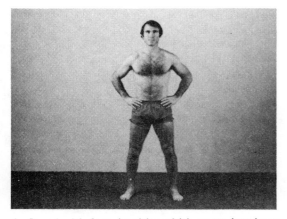

1. Stand with feet shoulder width apart, hands on your hips.

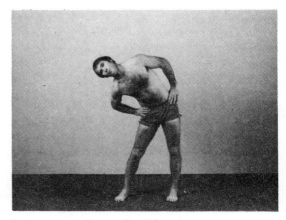

2. Begin rotating to the right.

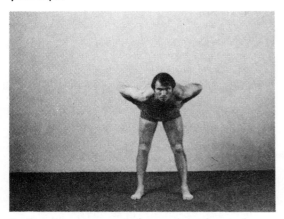

3. Continue the rotating movement forward . . .

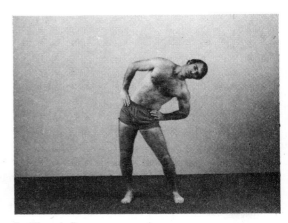

4. Then left . . .

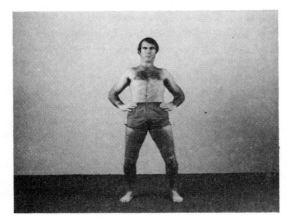

5. And back.

Hip Warm Up #2

Number of Repetitions
10
Physiological Benefits
This is an excellent exercise for the entire hip and waist area, loosening the spine, and increasing flexibility in the obliques, back, and abdomen. Upper leg muscles and tendons are also gently stressed.
Martial Arts Benefits
Strong, yet relaxed muscles are vital for delivering powerful kicks.
Pointers
It is very important to practice this exercise slowly. Do not jerk your body up too quickly—you don't want to wrench your spine. You should also concentrate on keeping your knees from bending during the exercise. Keep the weight on your feet evenly distributed. The shoulders should be relaxed and the arms outstretched throughout the entire exercise. You should be aware of keeping a steady and natural balance while developing the full range of motion to obtain the full benefits of this exercise.

Hip Warm Up #2

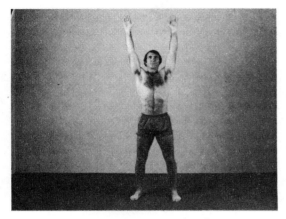

1. Raise your hands above your head.

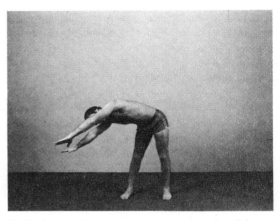

2. Begin rotating your upper torso to the right . . .

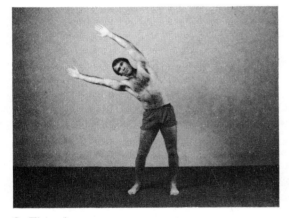

3. Then down.

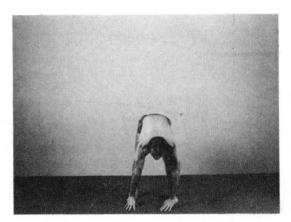

4. As you rotate forward, your fingers should brush the floor.

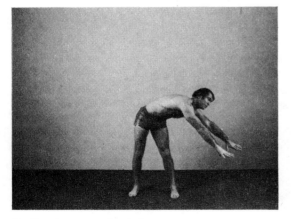

5. Continue rotating left.

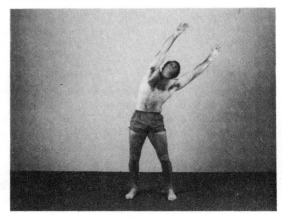

6. Then return to the upright position.

Waist Warm Up #1

If you do not have adequate flexibility in your waist, your upper torso will be immobile, your hips will be stiff, and your back and spine will be forced into rigid, unnatural postures.

Number of Repetitions

5-10 on each side

Physiological Benefits

This exercise strengthens and loosens the oblique, abdominal, and back muscles.

Martial Arts Benefits

Your balance, posture, and ability to lift your legs in the correct position for a kick will be improved.

Pointers

Concentrate on developing control when practicing this exercise. Don't jerk your legs or hyperextend your knee but try to keep your legs as straight as possible.

Waist Warm Up #1

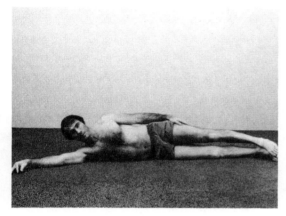

1. Lie on your right side, one hand extended for balance.

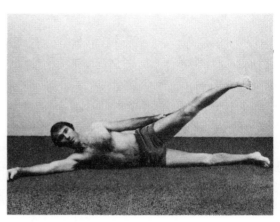

2. Begin raising your left leg.

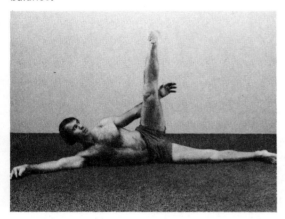

3. Continue raising it until you reach the point of tension. Hold, and return to the original position. Repeat on the opposite side.

Waist Warm Up #2

Number of Repetitions
5-10 on each side

Physiological Benefits
This exercise helps prevent tears in the thin sheets of muscles in your back. It also stretches out the oblique muscles, which tend to shorten and become stiff if not exercised regularly.

Martial Arts Benefits
When your waist is flexible, you can keep your upper body relatively immobile while moving your lower body. This helps you avoid telegraphing your movements to your opponent.

Pointers
Try to lift your body off the ground while raising your legs. This intensifies the stress placed on the oblique muscles. Avoid unnecessary strain and develop this exercise slowly.

Waist Warm Up #2

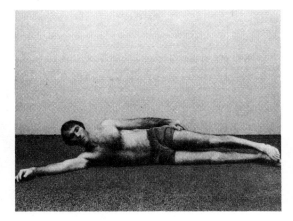

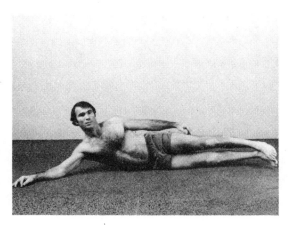

1. Lie on your right side, one arm extended for balance.

2. Bring legs and upper torso up as if trying to bring them together. You should feel tension in your waist.

Waist Warm Up #3

Waist exercises strengthen and loosen the oblique muscles, the lower back muscles, and the stomach muscles, all of which are vital for kicking.

Number of Repetitions
10

Physiological Benefits
Not only are all of the mid-body muscles strengthened, but the muscles holding the internal organs in place are also toned. Increased flexibility in this area will also improve the range of motion of the body's largest joint: the hip.

Martial Arts Benefits
All of the muscles affected by this exercise help you maintain the correct posture for kicking, and also helps strengthen the muscles used for the kicks themselves. A strong, flexible waist allows you to maneuver quickly and to bend at the waist to evade punches and kicks.

Pointers
Do not snap your body around too quickly in practicing this exercise, as this can pull lower back muscles or strain the abdominal muscles. Instead, begin exercising at a moderate pace, and then continue at a slightly faster pace once you have loosened up. Keep the legs straight, the chest open and shoulders relaxed and level.

Waist Warm Up #3

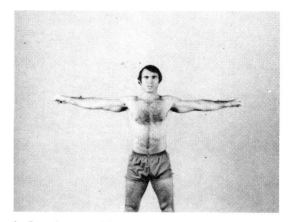

1. Stand erect with arms straight out at shoulder level.

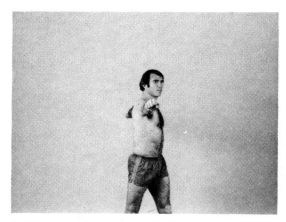

2. Turn your upper torso all the way to the left . .

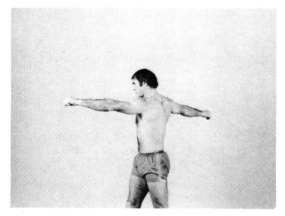

3. And all the way to the right.

Abdominal Warm Up #1

Strong abdominal muscles help the entire body stay toned. If these muscles are weak, it is easy to strain the back or leg muscles.

Number of Repetitions

5-10

Physiological Benefits

All of the abdominal muscles will be strengthened and toned by this exercise. The lower back muscles and upper thighs will also be stretched.

Martial Arts Benefits

When bringing the leg up for high kicks, strength in the abdominals can actually be more important than strength in the thigh muscles. A sheet of dense abdominal muscles also helps absorb the impact of hits or kicks to that area.

Pointers

Press up very slowly, and return to the original position equally slowly. Make sure you don't bounce, as that diminishes the effects of this exercise.

Abdominal Warm Up #1

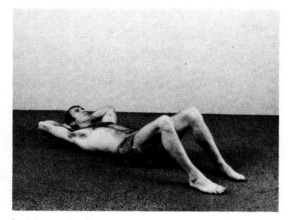

1. Lie on the floor with your knees bent, hands behind your head.

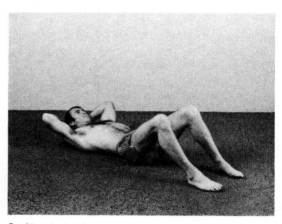

2. Slowly begin to curl up your upper torso.

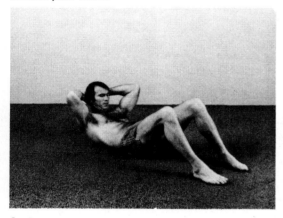

3. Continue curling until you reach the point of tension.

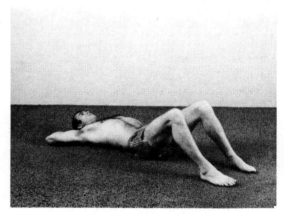

4. Hold, then slowly curl down.

Abdominal Warm Up #2

This exercise particularly concentrates on the lower abdominal muscles, which are often ignored.

Number of Repetitions

10-15

Physiological Benefits

In addition to strengthening the lower abdominal area, upper thigh, and lower back muscles, this exercise improves circulation in the legs.

Martial Arts Benefits

Endurance in kicking is enhanced when this exercise is practiced regularly.

Pointers

Keep your lower back flat on the floor and your feet flexed throughout the exercise. Don't jerk the legs or throw the knees out. Avoid unnecessary hyperextension of the legs and concentrate your efforts on the abdominals.

Abdominal Warm Up #2

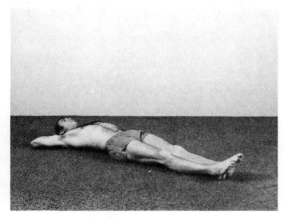

1. Lie flat on the floor.

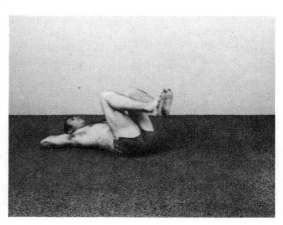

2. Bring both knees up to your chest.

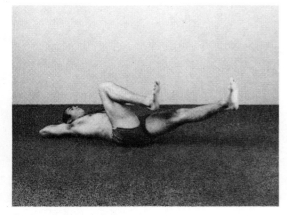

3. Extend the left leg.

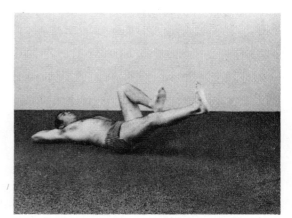

4. Retract the left leg, and at the same time extend the right leg. Continue this motion.

Abdominal Warm Up #3

Since strength can be built up in the abdominal muscles more quickly than in any other muscle group, you should be able to increase the number of counts for which you hold the extreme position in a short period of time.

Number of Repetitions

10

Physiological Benefits

This exercise strengthens the lower abdomen, back, upper thighs, calves (particularly when the toes are pointed), and gluteus muscles.

Martial Arts Benefits

In addition to the other benefits provided by abdominal exercises, this warm up focuses on improving your control. Control is vital when executing combinations as you need to fight the force of gravity which pulls your kicking leg down.

Pointers

Do not drop the legs quickly, but lower them with a slow, controlled motion. Make sure your feet are kept together throughout the exercise. In first starting out on this exercise, you may notice pressure in the small of your back. Proceed with this exercise gradually, avoid any back strain, and concentrate your mind on developing the abdominals. If the strain in the back continues, reduce the time the legs are held in the air or discontinue this exercise until a later date.

Abdominal Warm Up #3

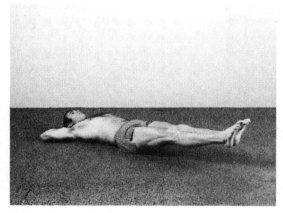

1. Lie flat on the floor.

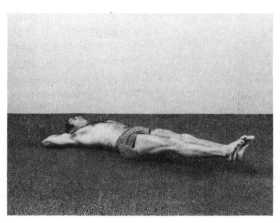

2. Begin raising both legs and hold them about six inches off the ground.

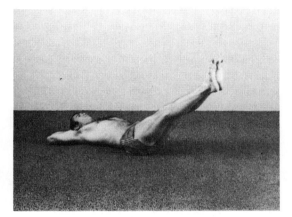

3. Raise both legs as high as possible and hold.

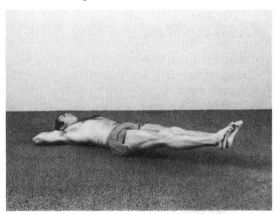

4. Slowly return the legs to the floor.

Back Warm Up #1

Practice back warm up exercises regularly to attain spinal flexibility and strong back muscles.

Number of Repetitions

5-10

Physiological Benefits

Flexibility of the spine and neck joint is accompanied by strength in the upper and lower back, abdomen, and chest.

Martial Arts Benefits

In loosening the upper body you will improve maneuvering, and help intensify the power of strikes and kicks.

Pointers

Be careful not to raise yourself past the point of tension. You must also avoid jerking your body up too quickly, as this can strain your back or pull your abdominal muscles. Keep the shoulders and chest relaxed. Do this exercise slowly and evenly.

Back Warm Up #1

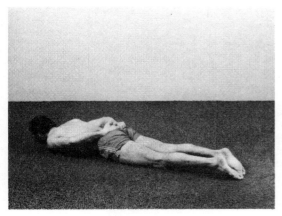

1. Lie flat on the floor on your stomach.

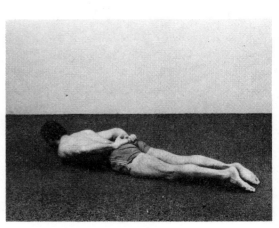

2. Begin lifting your upper torso.

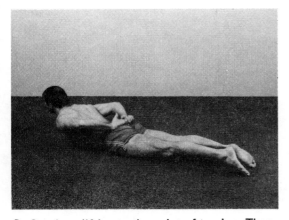

3. Continue lifting to the point of tension. Then hold.

Back Warm Up #2

Number of Repetitions
5-10
Physiological Benefits
This exercise provides a slow stretch of the upper and lower abdominals, loosens the spine, opens the front of the chest, and strengthens the thighs.
Martial Arts Benefits
Increased flexibility will improve your maneuvering.
Pointers
This exercise requires a slow rocking motion backwards and forwards. Be sure not to jerk your body. It is important to reach a completely relaxed state of mind and body to obtain the full benefits of this exercise.

Back Warm Up #2

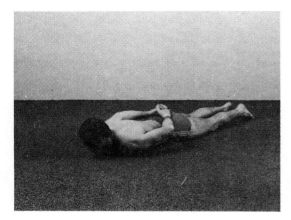

1. Lie flat on your stomach.

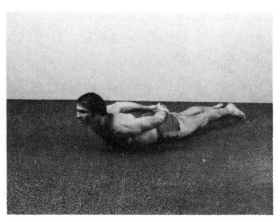

2. Lift your upper torso.

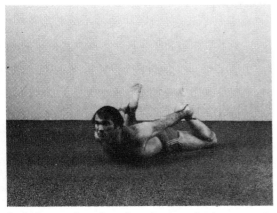

3. Lift your legs, bending them at the knees, and grab your ankles. Slowly rock back and forth before returning to the starting position.

Ankle Warm Up

Since the ankle is the joint which must bear the entire weight of the body, it tends to become strong but stiff. It is vital to keep this joint flexible in order to move quickly and execute powerful strikes with the foot.

Number of Repetitions

5-10

Physiological Benefits

By attaining the full range of motion of the ankles, you can help prevent sprains and strains, strengthen the arch, and improve the circulation in the foot. The front of the shin and the Achilles tendon in the back of the leg are also loosened.

Martial Arts Benefits

A flexible ankle helps position the foot properly for the different kicks. In a roundhouse kick, you need to flick the foot; in a heel and side kick, you must pull the foot back.

Pointers

Do not rotate the foot too quickly.

Ankle Warm Up

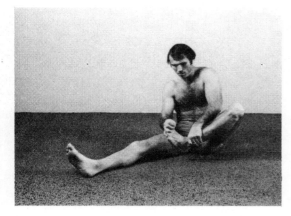

1. Sit on the floor with one leg extended straight in front of you. Grab the ankle of the left leg and pull it towards you.

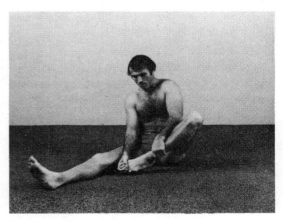

2. Rotate the foot down . . .

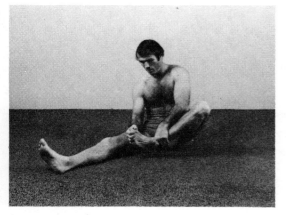

3. And around.

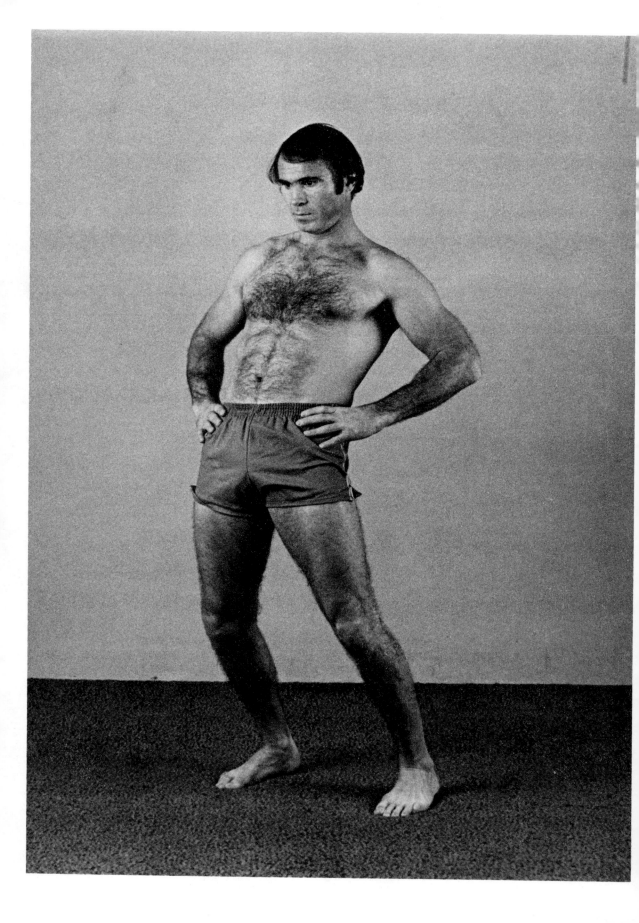

Upper Body Exercises

Exercises for the upper body concentrate on the muscles on the sides and back of the neck (trapezius), the shoulder muslces (deltoids), the upper back muscles (latissimus dorsi), the lower back muscles (lumbar muscles), the chest muscles (pectoralis major and minor), the abdominal muscles, and the waist (oblique) muscles. These muscle groups keep the body and head erect, hold the internal organs in place, and are used in raising, lowering and rotating the arms, head, and upper torso. As the back and neck muscles are especially subject to the stiffening effects of aging and stress, flexibility and strengthening exercises for these areas cannot be neglected. If you ever suffer from lower back pains, or have torn or wrenched back or neck muscles, you will want to pay careful attention to these exercises in your daily routine.

Neck Exercise

This exercise looks simple, but is one of the best ways of improving the overall flexibility of the neck and shoulders.

Number of Repetitions

Continue the exercise for as long as possible.

Physiological Benefits

Neck, shoulder, and upper back muscles are strengthened. The range of motion of the neck joint is also increased.

Martial Arts Benefits

If your neck does not have a full range of motion, you will absorb more of a punch's impact and can more easily be knocked out.

Pointers

Never jerk your head around, but practice the exercise with a slow, controlled motion. You should feel tension in the muscles, but no excessive pinching.

Neck Exercise

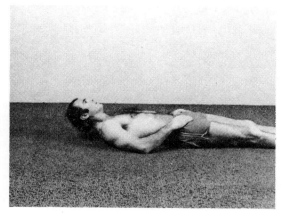

1. Lie flat on your back. Raise your head.

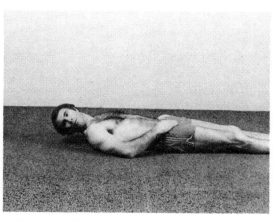

2. Turn it right . . .

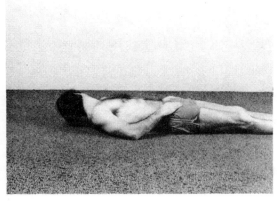

3. Then left.

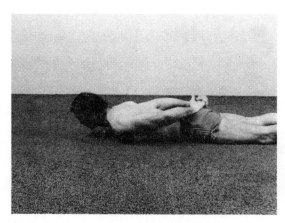

4. Roll over onto your stomach. Lift your head.

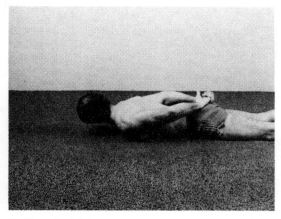

5. Turn it right . . .

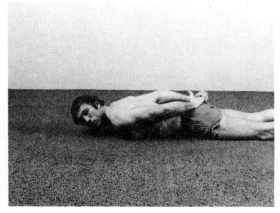

6. Then left.

Bridging Exercise #1

Bridging exercises concentrate on strengthening the neck and back muscles. This is particularly important in preventing spinal injuries.

Number of Repetitions

5-10

Physiological Benefits

This exercise stretches out the upper and lower abdominals, as well as the lower back and upper shoulder muscles. It strengthens the legs, neck, and back, and improves spinal flexibility.

Martial Arts Benefits

A strong neck is essential for absorbing or dodging blows to the head, as well as for executing head butts.

Pointers

Start very slowly when practicing this exercise. Be careful not to overarch or overtwist.

Bridging Exercise #1

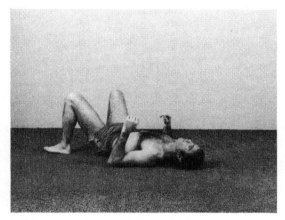

1. Lie on your back with knees bent.

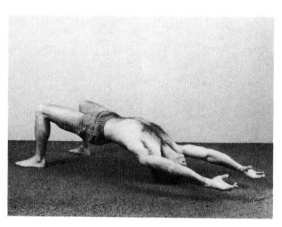

2. Arch your back and shift your body weight onto the crown of your head.

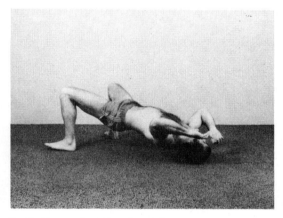

3. Roll your body to the right.

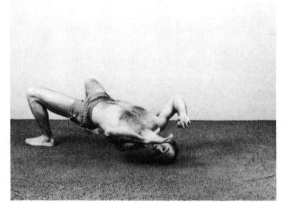

4. Roll your body to the left.

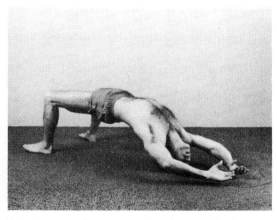

5. Return to the center and raise your body into a full arch.

Bridging Exercise #2

By strengthening these muscles you can prevent wrenching, twisting, or pulling the neck.

Number of Repetitions

5-10

Physiological Benefits

This exercise improves spinal flexibility while strengthening the neck muscles and back of the legs.

Martial Arts Benefits

The ability to roll with or evade blows to the head is enhanced.

Pointers

Practice this exercise with great control. Remember, the spine is delicate and can easily be damaged if you overextend the arch. It is always important to remember that these exercises should be developed gradually for lasting improvement. The body and mind should be naturally relaxed. Avoid unnecessary strain and tension. Do not hurry and always concentrate on the area of your body that you are exercising.

Bridging Exercise #2

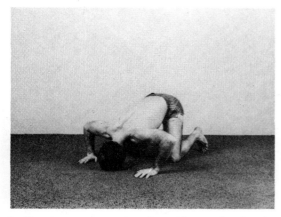

1. Get down on your hands and knees, forehead touching the floor.

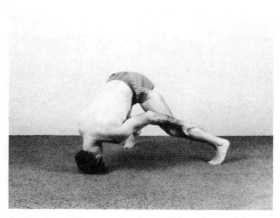

2. Begin to lift your body, shifting the weight onto your head.

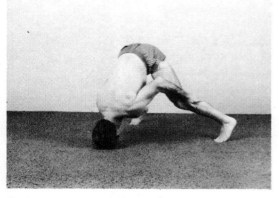

3. Rotate your neck forward . . .

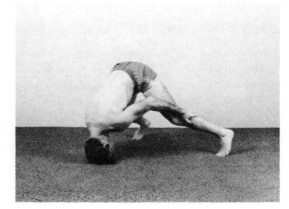

4. Right . . .

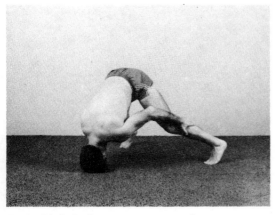

5. And left, before you return to the center.

Lower Back Stretch

This provides a nearly complete body stretch, as it affects the legs, groin muscle, chest muscles, and upper and lower back. If you do not overstretch when practicing this exercise, it is an excellent preparation for exercises which more fully concentrate on the lower back area.

Number of Repetitions

2-5

Physiological Benefits

In addition to providing a complete stretch of the legs and hips, this exercise requires you to arch the back for a stretch of all the lower back and lower abdominal muscles.

Martial Arts Benefits

Flexibility in the lower back is necessary for positioning the body correctly and for keeping the body from bouncing as you deliver the different types of kicks.

Pointers

Make sure that you brace yourself while practicing this exercise. Don't let yourself slip downwards too quickly, or pass your point of tension. With perseverance, patience and time you can develop your body to accomplish any type of exercise. Develop concentration and always keep a positive attitude. Once you have a negative thought or think that you cannot ever do the exercise, you have already lost half of the battle. Always remember that discipline is a state of mind as well as the process of training.

Lower Back Stretch

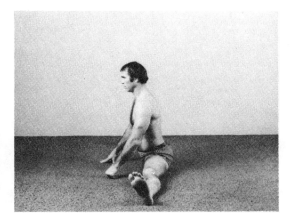

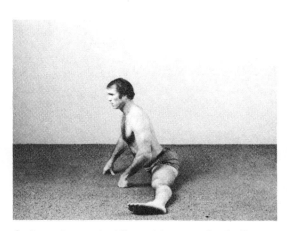

1. Assume the Chinese splits position.

2. Lean forward while arching your back. Brace yourself with your arms.

Lower Back Exercise #1

Strength does not come from rigidity, but from relaxed muscles. To contract with maximum power, the muscles must first be completely loose and well conditioned.

Number of Repetitions

10-15

Physiological Benefits

This exercise stretches out the lower back and the hamstrings. It also increases circulation in the legs.

Martial Arts Benefits

Flexibility in the lower back and legs is necessary for kicking, maneuvering, and footwork.

Pointers

Don't strain or bounce in this exercise. You should feel a gentle stretch and relaxation of the muscles.

Lower Back Exercise #1

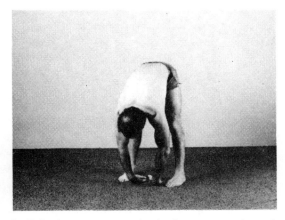

1. Relaxing your upper body, lean over and touch the floor.

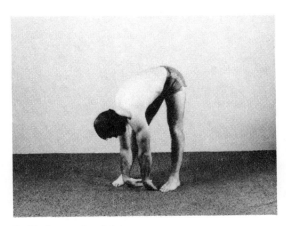

2. Twist to the right . . .

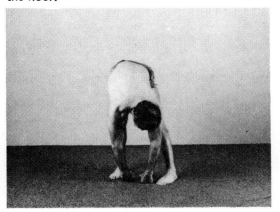

3. Then left.

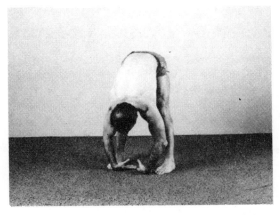

4. Relax and drop your body as low as possible.

Lower Back Exercise #2

The sheet of muscles across the lower back is rarely stretched out, but it is vital in all movements. The tighter your lower back muscles have become, the less maneuverability your upper torso will have.

Number of Repetitions

5-10

Physiological Benefits

This exercise stretches and relaxes the lower back muscles, the lower abdomen, and the legs. Spinal flexibility is also improved.

Martial Arts Benefits

You will have greater ease in maintaining an erect posture for delivering kicks.

Pointers

Don't bounce or overstrain when practicing this exercise, as it is very easy to tear the back muscles. Always concentrate on the muscle group you are exercising.

Lower Back Exercise #2

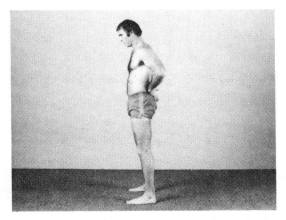

1. Stand erect, hands resting on your lower back.

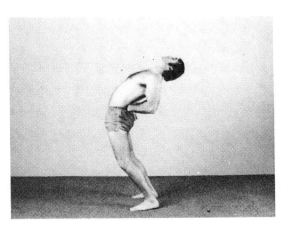

2. Lean backwards as far as possbile.

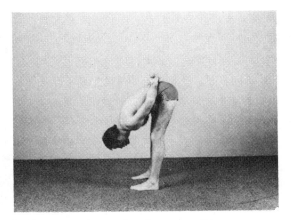

3. Then lean forward as far as possible.

Shoulders and Chest Exercise

This exercise is excellent for loosening the shoulders and chest while strengthening the arms, chest, and back muscles.

Number of Repetitions
5-10

Physiological Benefits
In addition to loosening and strengthening the upper torso, this exercise increases the range of motion in the shoulders.

Martial Arts Benefits
It is necessary to be relaxed to block effectively and to snap your techniques. Maneuverability is also enhanced.

Pointers
Do not pass the point of tension when practicing this exercise. When you are executing the backwards movement, be careful to avoid straining the shoulder muscles.

Shoulders and Chest Exercise

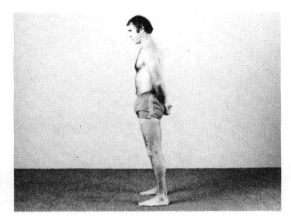

1. Clasp your hands behind your back.

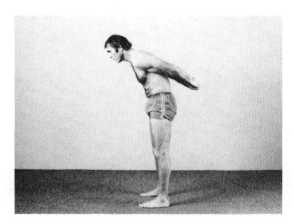

2. Lift your clasped hands.

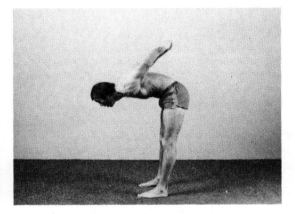

3. When you have raised them to the point of tension, begin bending over.

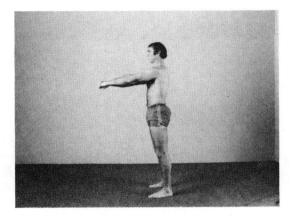

4. Clasp your hands in front of your body.

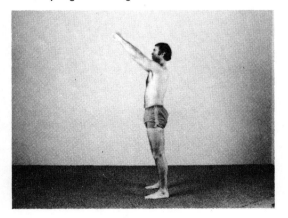

5. Begin lifting your hands.

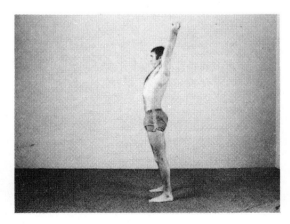

6. Pull them behind your head.

Waist and Abdomen Exercise

The steady, controlled movement of the hip joint helps tone the muscles holding the internal organs in position.

Number of Repetitions

10-20 in each direction

Physiological Benefits

This exercise stretches and relaxes the lower back, hips, spine, and lower pelvic region.

Martial Arts Benefits

A loose waist, hips, and strong abdominals are essential for fast, powerful kicks.

Pointers

Don't move too rapidly or make too large circles. You must avoid building up too much pressure on the sides of the legs. Maintain a smooth and constant rotational movement with easy changes in direction from right to left and left to right.

Waist and Abdomen Exercise

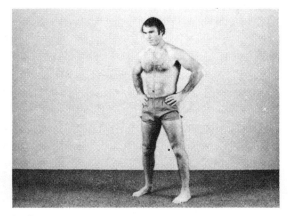

1. Stand erect with feet shoulder width apart, hands on hip.

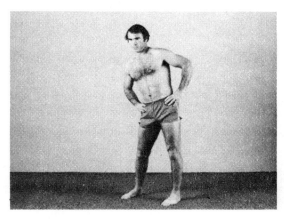

2. Begin rotating your hips to the left.

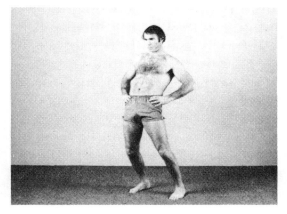

3. Continue the rotation forward . . .

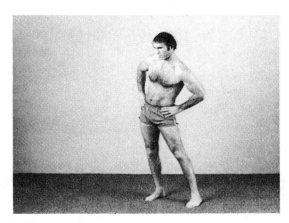

4. Right . . .

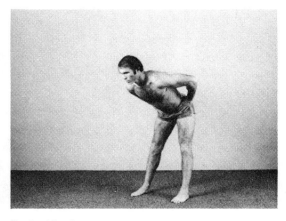

5. And back.

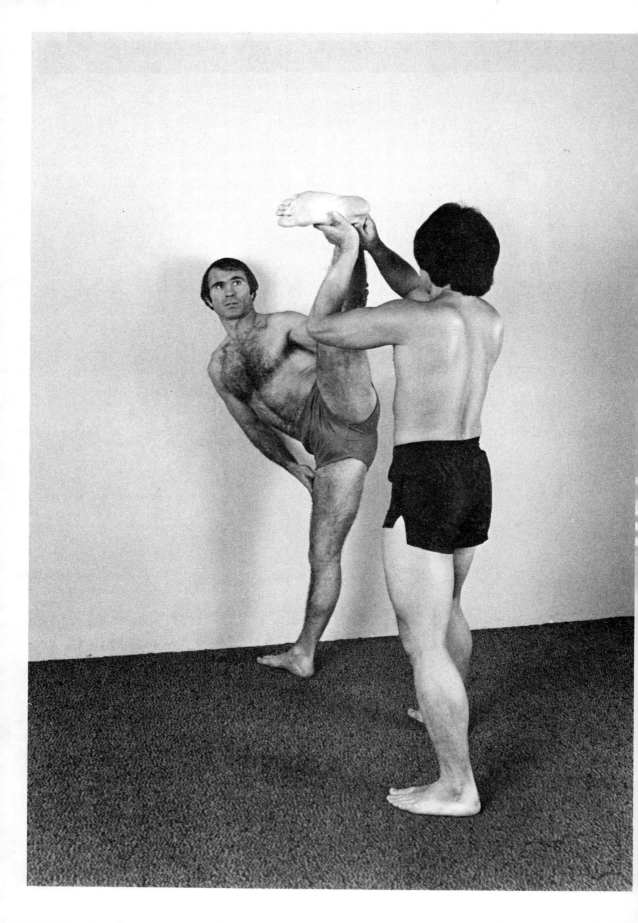

Lower Body Exercises

For flexbility in the legs, hips, and groin area, you must work the sartorius, or hamstring muscles, the quadriceps muscle in the upper thigh, the biceps fermoris muscle in the back of the upper leg, and the gastrocnemius or calf muscle. Flexibility also depends on having a complete range of motion in the knee, ankle and hip joints. Although the following exercises for these areas range from beginning to very advanced, the beginner can try almost every exercise if he is careful to perform each one at his own level. Make sure you stretch only to the point of tension, hold at that point, relax, and then return to your maximum stretch. Through slow, steady stretching you will be able to achieve the more advanced positions.

Knee Bends #1

Full knee bends can be very damaging to the knees. When performing any exercise that stresses the knee joint, you must be very careful not to put too much pressure on this easily damaged joint. Never continue with an exercise after a joint is in pain.

Number of Repetitions
10

Physiological Benefits
This exercise strengthens the upper thighs, the muscles supporting the knees, and the calf muscles. It also helps improve your balance.

Martial Arts Benefits
This is an excellent exercise to improve your kicking, as it strengthens both the standing leg and the muscles used to raise the knee.

Pointers
Practice this exercise as slowly as possible, in order to maximally increase your strength. Be sure not to drop your body all the way down. Try to keep your body as erect as possible throughout the entire exercise—do not lean forward to help you resume a standing position. In addition to strengthening the knee, this exercise also develops balance. Concentrate on your posture as well as the knees.

Knee Bends #1

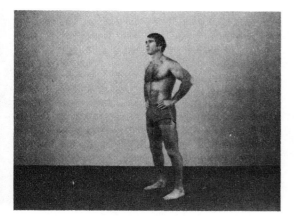

1. Stand erect with feet shoulder width apart.

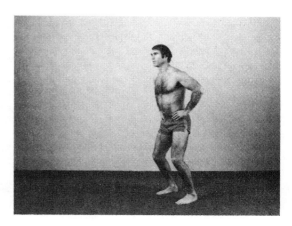

2. Slowly begin to bend your knees.

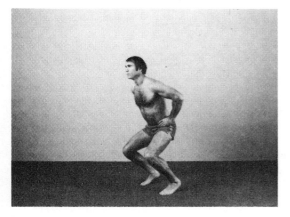

3. Continue bending until you are halfway down.

Knee Bends #2

Number of Repetitions
10 to 15 in each direction
Physiological Benefits
This exercise concentrates on developing a complete range of motion in the knee joints. It is also excellent for loosening the ankles.
Martial Arts Benefits
Loose knees help you to snap your kicks, and to avoid the problems that come from hyperextending this joint. Foot maneuvering for evasion is also improved.
Pointers
Make sure you do not put your hands directly on the knee caps, as it is easy to push the knee cap out of its proper position. Avoid building up any sideways pressure on the knees. The body should be kept erect throughout the exercise. In doing this exercise for the first time, you may feel a slight pull in the Achilles tendon, indicating that this area also does not have proper conditioning.

Knee Bends #2

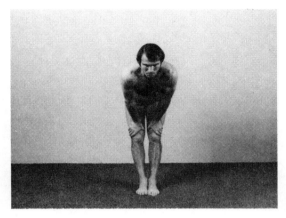

1. Stand with feet together, hands on your knees.

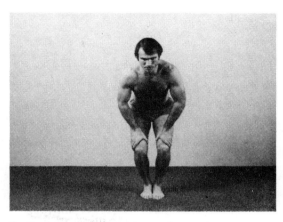

2. Begin rotating your knees forward . . .

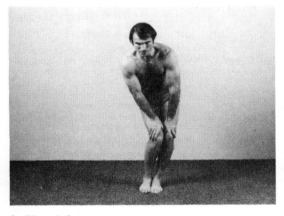

3. Then left . . .

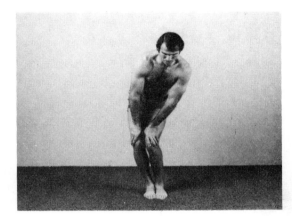

4. Then right.

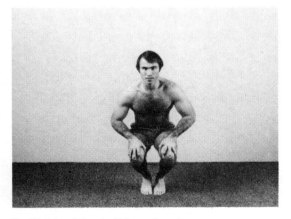

5. Finish with a half knee bend.

Toe Touch

The lower back and leg muscles are the first muscles of the body to become tight as you age. If these muscles are not loosened regularly, the tightening process will eventually make walking and even sitting up difficult.

Number of Repetitions
5-10

Physiological Benefits
This exercise stretches all of the lower back and leg muscles, loosening the hamstrings, tendons in the back of the knees, and lower back muscles. The neck muscles are also given a gentle stretch.

Martial Arts Benefits
You need maximum flexibility in the back and leg muscles for high, powerful kicks.

Pointers
Never bounce when practicing this exercise. Don't hunch your back; it should be as flat as possible throughout the exercise. The legs should be straight with knees locked.

Toe Touch

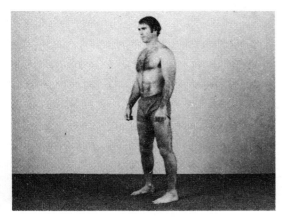

1. Stand erect, feet shoulder width apart.

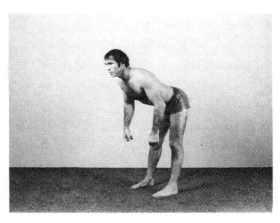

2. Begin bending over, keeping your back flat.

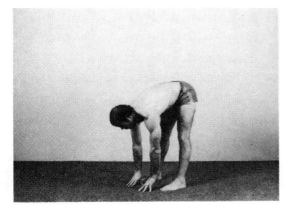

3. Continue bending until your fingers touch the floor.

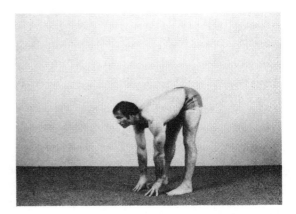

4. Then look up and slightly arch your back to stretch the lower back muscles.

Calf and Torso Stretch

Unless you specifically exercise the calf, these muscles may not be given the strengthening and loosening necessary for full, powerful movements of the lower leg, foot, and ankle.

Number of Repetitions

5-10

Physiological Benefits

In addition to stretching and strengthening the calves, upper thighs, and abdominals, this exercise will also strengthen your arches and improve your balance.

Martial Arts Benefits

A strong base leg and powerful snappy kicks require strong calf muscles and flexible ankles. Good balance is also vital in executing a series of kicks.

Pointers

Make sure that your feet do not turn outward or sag during the exercise. Try to keep your muscles tight while rising.

Calf and Torso Stretch

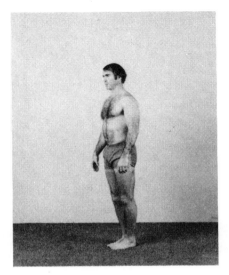

1. Stand erect with feet together.

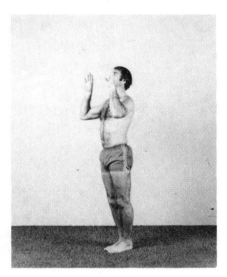

2. Begin lifting your arms.

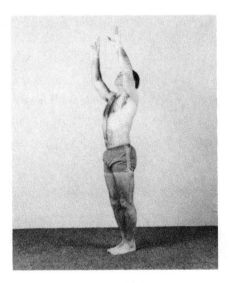

3. Reach upwards as high as possible, feeling the stretch in your arms and abdominal muscles.

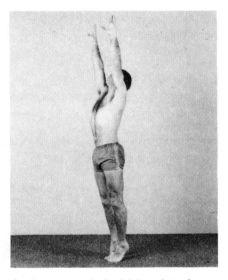

4. As you reach the high point of your stretch, come up on your toes.

Sartorious Exercise

The sartorius (hamstrings) and the Achilles tendons must be flexible for maintaining balance as well as for delivering kicks.

Number of Repetitions
5-10 on each side

Physiological Benefits
This exercise stretches all of the tendons and ligaments in the legs, as well as providing a gentle stretch of the leg muscles.

Martial Arts Benefits
Loosened tendons in the leg allow you to maintain and easily regain your balance, as well as to deliver effective kicks.

Pointers
Make sure you don't rock too vigorously while practicing this exercise. Carefully regulate the pressure on the bent knees.

Sartorius Exercise

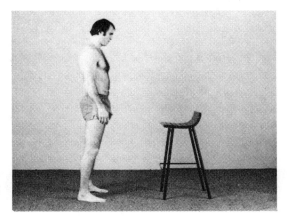

1. Stand two feet from a table or chair.

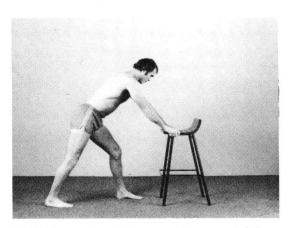

2. Hold onto the chair as you bring your left leg forward.

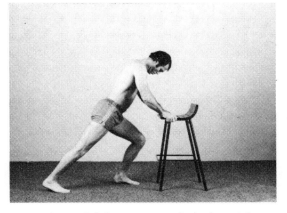

3. Bend your left knee to stretch the hamstrings of your right leg.

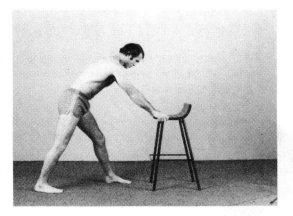

4. Rock back and forth to gently increase the stretch.

Biceps Femoris Exercise #1

Men often have more difficulties than women in keeping the legs stretched out and flexible. It is important to work the muscles, tendons, and ligaments of the leg every day.

Number of Repetitions

10-15

Physiological Benefits

This exercise stretches the lower back, hamstrings, and tendons behind the knees.

Martial Arts Benefits

Smooth, fast kicks which do not overstrain the knee or hamstrings require stretched muscles and loosened tendons.

Pointers

Begin practicing this exercise slowly, and do not stretch past the point of tension. Never jerk or bounce. Eventually, you should be able to reach your chest to your leg. Your chin may be on or past your knee. Maintain good balance in the legs and keep your breathing even.

Biceps Femoris Exercise #1

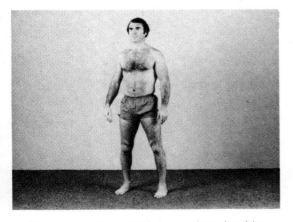

1. Stand erect, feet slightly more than shoulder width apart.

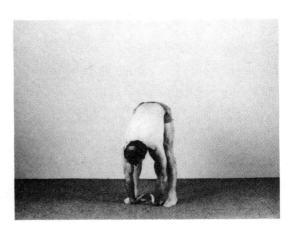

2. Lean over, touching the backs of your hands on the floor.

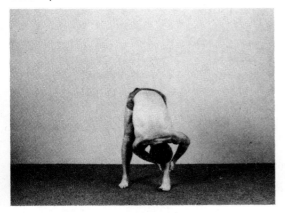

3. Grab your left ankle. Pull your head to your left knee.

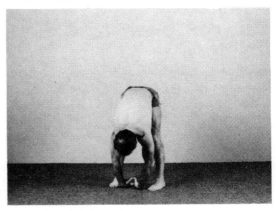

4. Return to the center.

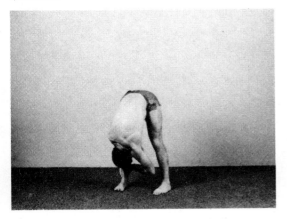

5. Then grab your right ankle and pull your head to the right knee.

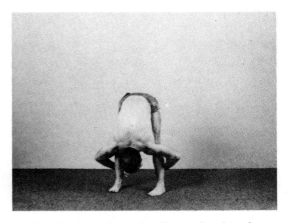

6. Grab both ankles and pull your head to the centerline.

Biceps Femoris Exercise #2

This exercise provides a more vigorous stretch of the same muscle groups affected by Biceps Femoris Exercise #1, and should not be practiced until the sufficient degree of flexibility has been attained.

Number of Repetitions

5-10

Physiological Benefits

Because this exercise is more strenuous, it also helps in opening the hips.

Martial Arts Benefits

This exercise improves balance, kicking, and overall mobility.

Pointers

Be sure you practice slowly and carefully so as not to lose your balance. Your feet should be stable throughout the exercise, and you should be able to keep your ankles from twisting. It helps to concentrate on the twisting motion of the waist.

Biceps Femoris Exercise #2

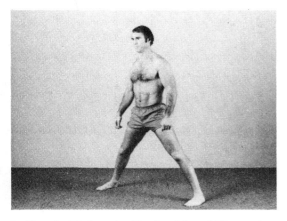

1. Stand with legs double shoulder width apart.

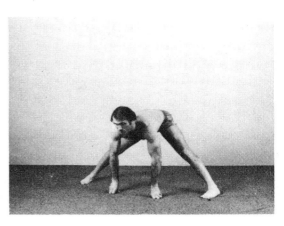

2. Lean down, touching your hands to the floor.

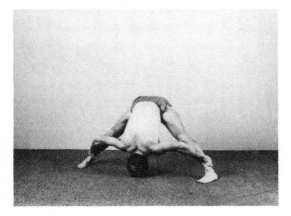

3. Grab your ankles and pull your head down to touch the centerline.

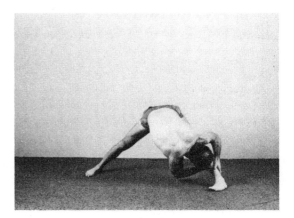

4. Then grab your left ankle, pulling your head to your left shin.

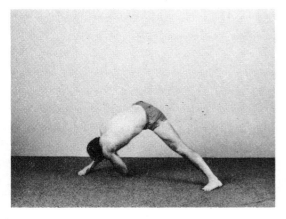

5. Grab your right ankle, pulling your head to the right shin.

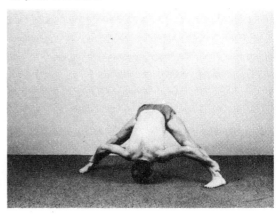

6. Return to the centerline.

Biceps Femoris Exercise #3

Anyone can eventually learn to perform a complete side split. However, it is essential to begin practicing this exercise very slowly and gradually, and not to move past the point of tension. Let gravity help you achieve a good stretch. Remember, it is very easy to pull groin muscles.

Number of Repetitions

2-5

Physiological Benefits

This exercise stretches the inside of the thigh, the hamstring, and all of the muscles and tendons in the hip. The ankles are gently stretched and loosened.

Martial Arts Benefits

Flexibility in the groin muscles is important for all kicks. Strong ankles will improve stability in kicking and in delivering other techniques.

Pointers

The back foot should be turned on the instep so your leg and ankle will be stretched. When you rock forward, keep your chest flat. Be sure to brace yourself with your arms when you first start practicing the exercise.

Biceps Femoris Exercise #3

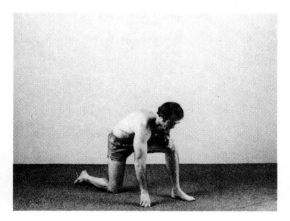

1. Bend your right knee, lowering it to the floor.

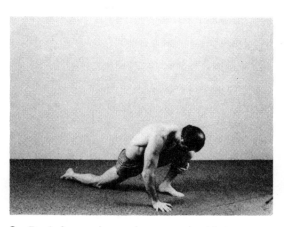

2. Rock forward, pressing your chest into your left leg.

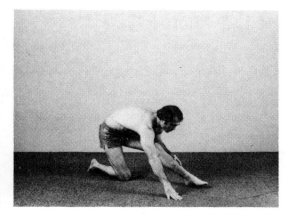

3. Rock backwards, keeping your back stretched.

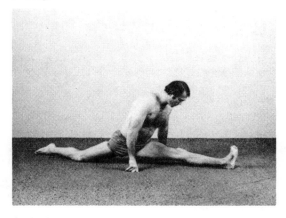

4. Slide your left leg forward into a splits position. You should feel tension in your groin muscles.

Leg Stretch #1

This exercise is excellent for stretching all of the leg, groin, and hip muscles. It is possible to get a greater degree of stretch from this exercise than from performing a similar exercise on the floor.

Number of Repetitions

5

Physiological Benefits

As mentioned above, the thigh muscles, hamstrings, and hip muscles are thoroughly stretched out in this exercise. It is also good for improving balance and control.

Martial Arts Benefits

This is an ideal exercise for improving your kicks. It helps in developing balance and stability needed for standing on one leg while delivering powerful kicks with the other.

Pointers

Make sure your partner does not drop too quickly. Speed is not important in this exercise. Develop this exercise gradually. Your partner should be concentrating on helping you develop your ability. Your partner should feel you stretch as you are stretching yourself. It is dangerous to do exercises with a partner who is not awake and aware. Exercising with a partner will help you greatly but both partners must be working towards the same goal and participate equally in helping each other. This not only enhances the exercise, but makes the exercise interesting and different.

Leg Stretch #1

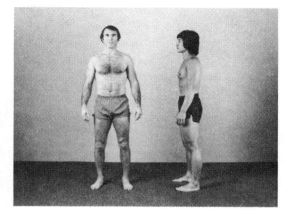

1. Stand erect with left side towards your partner.

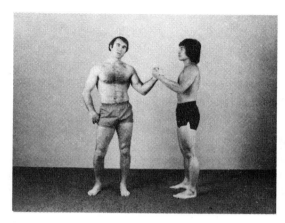

2. Grab his hand for support.

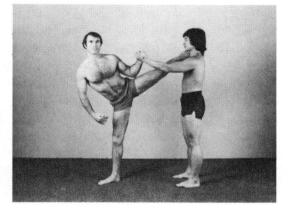

3. Put your left leg on his right shoulder.

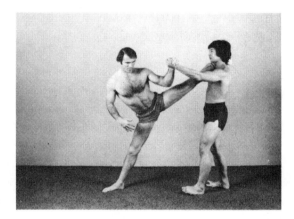

4. Relax as your partner slowly moves back.

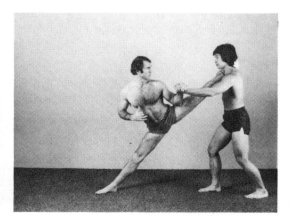

5. Tell your partner to stop at the point of tension. Hold for 30 seconds.

Leg Stretch #2

Number of Repetitions
5
Physiological Benefits
This exercise focuses on stretching the inner thigh and groin muscles. The wall braces you and prevents your body from moving to relieve the pressure of the stretch.
Martial Arts Benefits
This stretch helps provide the flexibility necessary for kicking.
Pointers
Be sure to practice this exercise very slowly. Do not go beyond the point of tension. Be patient, and your legs will gradually loosen up. Always remember that lasting results are developed gradually. The awareness and sensitivity of both partners cannot be overly stressed. Both partners should be working to develop each other.

Leg Stretch #2

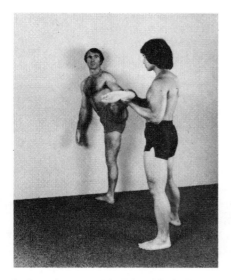

1. Stand erect with right side facing the wall. Your partner holds your left leg.

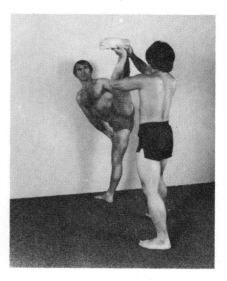

2. Your partner begins pushing up on your leg.

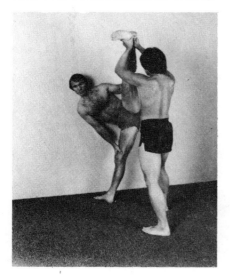

3. Relax as your partner continues the pressure.

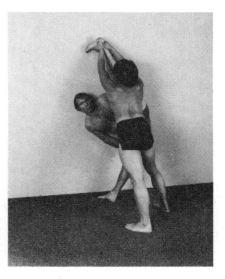

4. Eventually your foot should touch the wall.

Leg Stretch #3
Forward Push

As this leg stretch is practiced from a different angle than the previous two, it affects different muscles. All muscle groups in the legs must be stretched to attain complete flexibility.

Number of Repetitions

5

Physiological Benefits

This exercise works the inner thigh, groin muscles, waist and hip area, and strengthens the ankles.

Martial Arts Benefits

The movement in this exercise is similar to that used in the roundhouse kick.

Pointers

Don't move beyond the point of tension. Stay as erect as possible during the exercise, and avoid hunching the body. Don't expect to have sufficient flexibility to put your foot against the wall when you first start practicing this exercise. Concentrate on the muscles you are stretching and do not forget about balance even though you are using a wall.

Leg Stretch #3—Forward Push

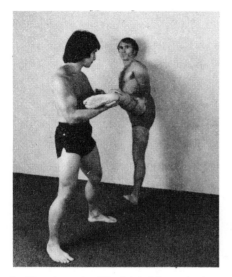

1. Stand erect with right side against the wall.

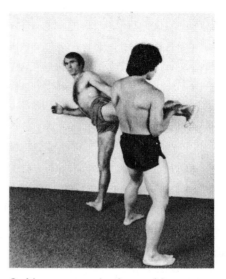

2. Your partner begins pushing your leg towards the wall.

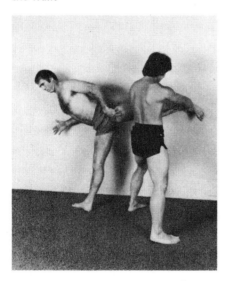

3. Tell your partner to stop at the point of tension.

Leg Stretch #4
Backwards Push

Number of Repetitions
5
Physiological Benefits
This exercise stretches the waist, hip, inner thigh, and groin muscles, and strengthens the leg muscles and ankles.
Martial Arts Benefits
Flexibility in the legs and hips helps prepare your leg to kick or block an attack.
Pointers
Avoid putting undue pressure on your knee. It is very easy to overstretch and strain the groin muscles in this exercise.

Leg Stretch #4—Backwards Push

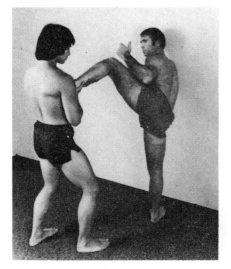

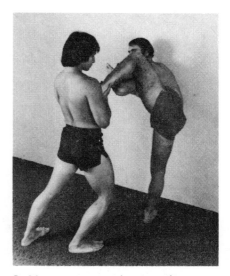

1. Stand erect, with right side against the wall, Your partner holds your leg with the knee bent.

2. Your partner pushes your leg, bending the knee furtner.

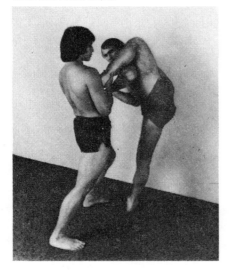

3. Slide your shoulder under the knee to bring the knee as close to the wall as possible.

Leg Stretch #5

Number of Repetitions
5
Physiological Benefits
This exercise stretches the inner thigh, lower stomach, lower back, and back of the legs.
Martial Arts Benefits
This leg stretch is particularly valuable in preparing you for a high, powerful side kick.
Pointers
Reach forward with your chest, rather than hunching your back. Make sure your partner doesn't push too fast or too hard.

Leg Stretch #5

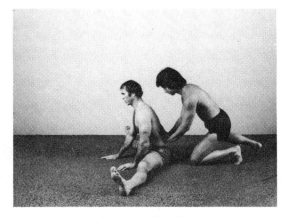

1. Sit with your legs spread as far apart as possible, Your partner begins pushing on your lower back.

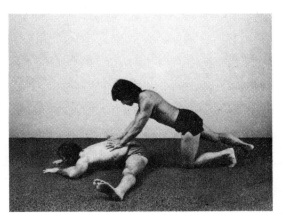

2. Your partner continues to apply steady pressure on your back, pushing you forward.

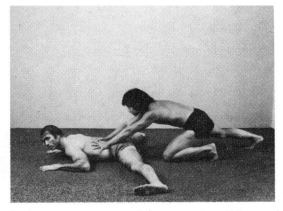

3. As your partner continues to push, roll forward slightly, bringing your chest flat on the floor.

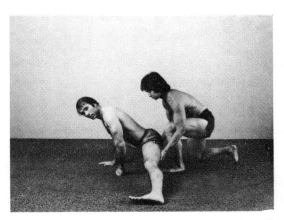

4. If you are unable to bring your upper torso all the way to the floor, have your partner support your thighs.

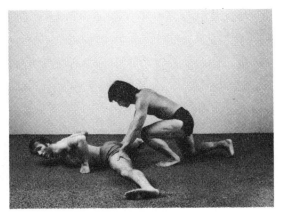

5. From this position roll down to the floor.

Leg Stretch #6

The best exercise for improving the side kick is actually practicing the side kick. That is what you will essentially be doing in this exercise. However, you will be able to increase the number of times you can repeat the kick by supporting your leg with your hands.

Number of Repetitions

5-15

Physiological Benefits

Balance and control is enhanced, hip flexibility is improved, and the ankles, waist, and inner thigh muscles are strengthened.

Martial Arts Benefits

Although the side kick particularly benefits from the diligent practice of this exercise, your overall strength and control in executing any of the kicks will be improved.

Pointers

Don't hyperextend your leg or let the ankle of the base leg wobble. Stand as erect as possible, and keep your body from dropping as you continue the kicking movement. Concentrate on balance and extension.

Leg Stretch #6

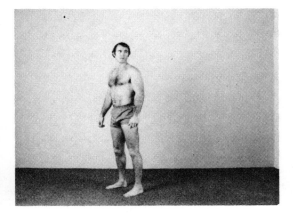

1. Stand erect, two feet from the wall.

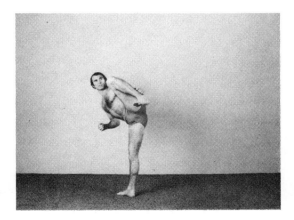

2. Bring your left knee up.

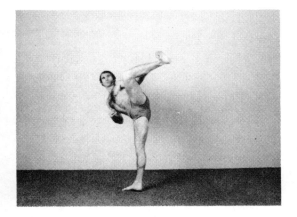

3. Using your arm for support, begin to extend your left leg.

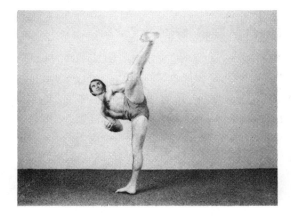

4. Extend your leg out fully, and hold before returning it to the cocked position.

Pancake Stretch

This stretch of the inner thigh muscles is less radical than the splits, and is good for a beginner.

Number of Repetitions

5-10

Physiological Benefits

This exercise loosens the ankles, tendons and ligaments in the knee, and hip area. It also stretches the inner thigh and groin muscles.

Martial Arts Benefits

It is important to keep the hips loose for powerful kicks. You need flexibility in the foot and ankle in order to maintain the different foot positions required for the various kicks.

Pointers

Keep the back erect while practicing this exercise. Exert steady pressure on your knees rather than bouncing them downward. Eventually, both knees will easily touch the floor.

Pancake Stretch

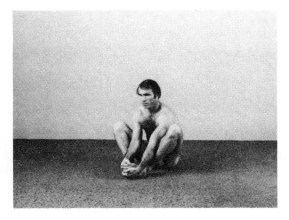

1. Sit on the floor, knees bent, soles of the feet touching.

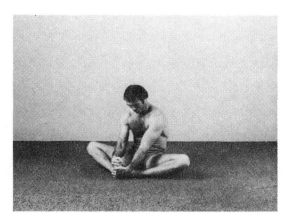

2. Apply pressure to your knees, trying to push them as close to the floor as possible.

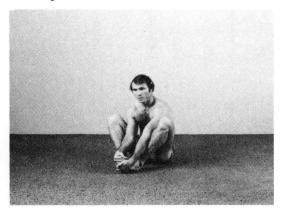

3. Relax the pressure, returning to the original position.

Splits–Advanced

This advanced exercise should be attempted only if you are already extremely flexible in the groin and leg muscles.

Number of Repetitions

5

Physiological Benefits

This exercise stretches the legs, inner thigh, and hip areas. The lower back and abdominal muscles are also loosened.

Martial Arts Benefits

By achieving the flexibility to execute very high kicks, your lower kicks will have substantially more power. A high degree of leg flexibility also improves your skill in footwork.

Pointers

Since this exercise provides an extreme stretch, you must carefully watch the amount of tension you allow to build up. Increase the degree of stretch very slowly. Again, as for every exercise, patience and diligence are of utmost importance.

Splits—Advanced

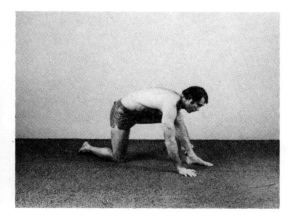

1. Lower yourself onto your right knee.

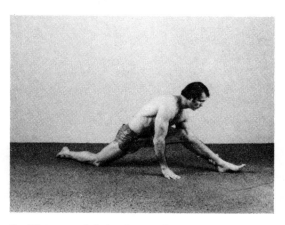

2. Slide your left leg forward.

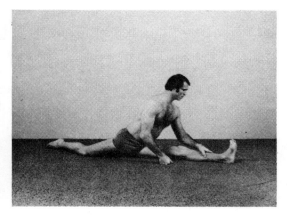

3. Assume the splits position.

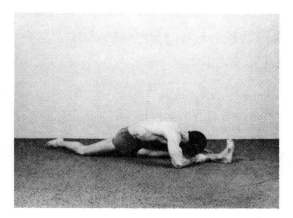

4. Lower your chest to your leg.

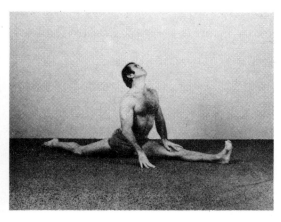

5. Arch backwards, stretching your abdominal muscles.

Chinese Splits

This is a very advanced exercise that provides a radical stretch to the leg muscles. Do not expect to achieve a complete split immediately.

Number of Repetitions

2-3

Physiological Benefits

This exercise stretches the hips, inner thigh, and groin muscles. It also loosens the ankles. When the upper torso is angled forward, the lower back will also be stretched.

Martial Arts Benefits

This exercise systematically stretches all of the muscles required for high, snappy kicks. It also gives you the flexibility needed for smooth, quick footwork.

Pointers

Control is very important in this exercise. Do not allow your body to sink too fast. Do not stretch past the point of tension, or you may pull a groin muscle. It is also important not to push on your kneecaps with your hands, as it is easy to slide the kneecaps out of position. This is an advanced but not an impossible exercise. If you feel that you will never be able to accomplish this exercise, you have the wrong attitude about training. If you have too much confidence and expect quick results, you do not understand the meaning of discipline. Develop gradually, concentrate on mastering this exercise with patience and perseverance.

Chinese Splits

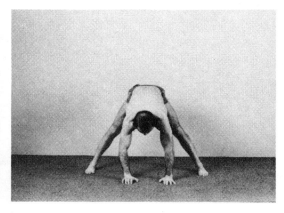

1. Lean over, touching your palms to the floor.

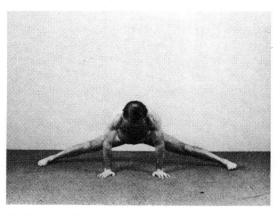

2. Begin sliding your legs out, bracing yourself with your arms.

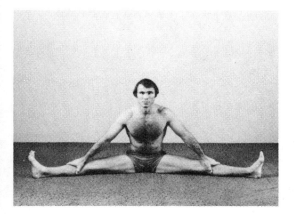

3. Put your hands on your knees and flex the toes upwards.

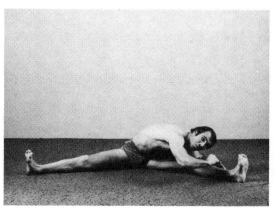

4. Pull your chest to your left leg . . .

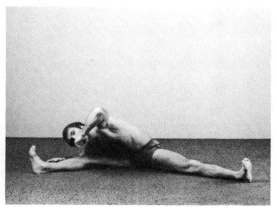

5. Then to your right leg.

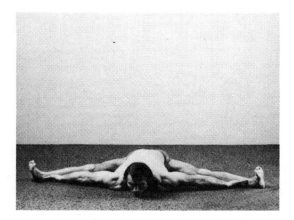

6. Finally, pull your body to the centerline before returning to the upright position.

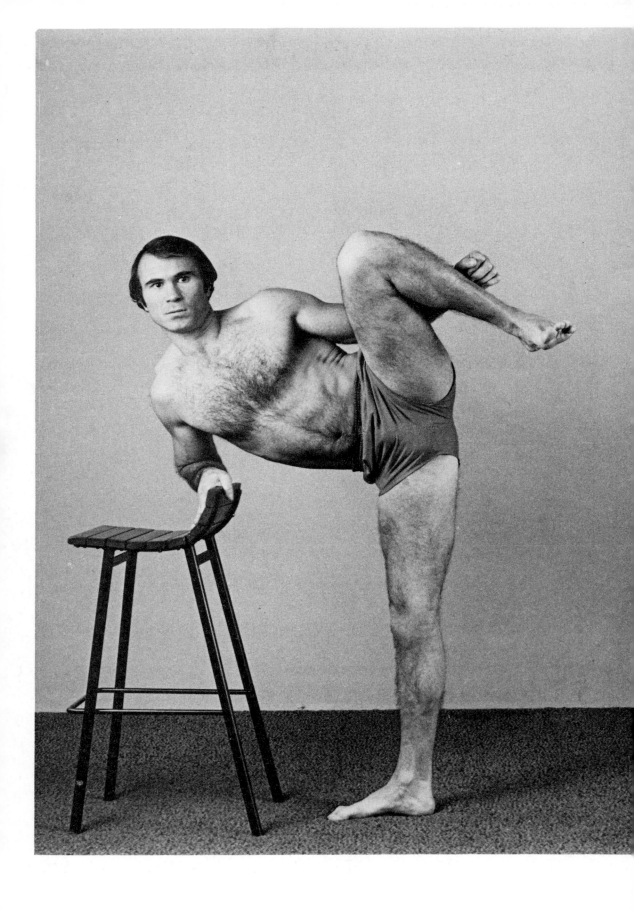

Balance Exercises

Good balance is the basis of all physical activities. In the martial arts, it is imperative to have superb balance in order to deliver techniques effectively. Many people believe that one must be born with a good sense of balance, and that it cannot be learned. This is untrue. Through patience and perseverance, anyone can improve their sense of balance.

When you begin these exercises, you may find that at first you will constantly have to support yourself, or you may need to extend your arms to regain your balance. Feel free to do this in the beginning stages. Eventually, you will not need these aids.

There are several techniques which will help you maintain your balance. Throughout the exercise, focus your eyes on a single point. This helps provide stability. You should also concentrate on relaxing. If you feel yourself losing balance, relax your muscles and breathe slowly and evenly.

Once you can maintain your balance in these exercises, begin to experiment with variations that will continually test and improve your balance. For example, try the balance exercises with your eyes closed.

Balance Exercise #1

Supporting yourself on a chair allows you to concentrate on developing the muscles required for kicking without concerning yourself with your balance. However, as you begin to acquire stability, use the chair only as an aid if you feel yourself losing your balance. Eventually, you will be able to practice this exercise using no prop at all.

Number of Repetitions

10-15

Physiological Benefits

This exercise provides a total stretch of the legs. It also loosens the waist, lower back, and hips, while improving your balance.

Martial Arts Benefits

Balance adds power, speed, focus, and control to all martial arts techniques. Exercises of this sort help develop these necessary qualities.

Pointers

If you lose your balance, be careful not to fall on the chair. Don't hyperextend your leg. Do not develop a mental dependence on the chair. Even with support, you must always concentrate on developing a sense of balance throughout your body and in the movement you are executing.

Balance Exercise #1

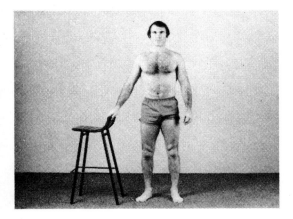

1. Hold onto the chair.

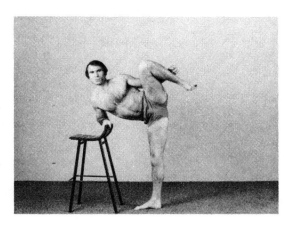

2. Bring your left knee up as high as possible.

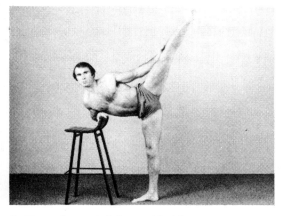

3. Extend your left leg and hold.

Balance Exercise #2

This exercise should be practiced without the supporting chair as soon as possible.

Number of Repetitions

10-15

Physiological Benefits

This exercise stretches the lower abdomen, back, and upper thigh. It also improves leg control.

Martial Arts Benefits

When you increase your leg control, you can place your kicks more precisely. This exercise also improves ankle stability and body positioning.

Pointers

Make sure you extend the leg with a slow, controlled motion.

Balance Exercise #2

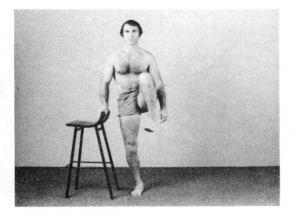

1. Holding onto a chair, bring your left knee up in front of you.

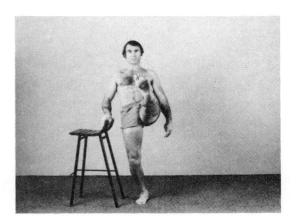

2. Extend the leg forward.

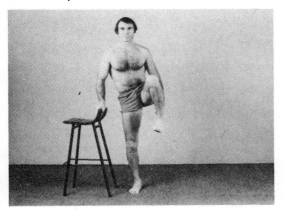

3. Return to the bent position . . .

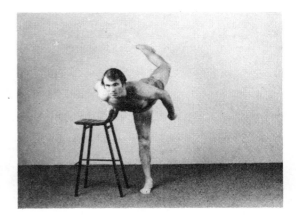

4. And extend the leg behind you.

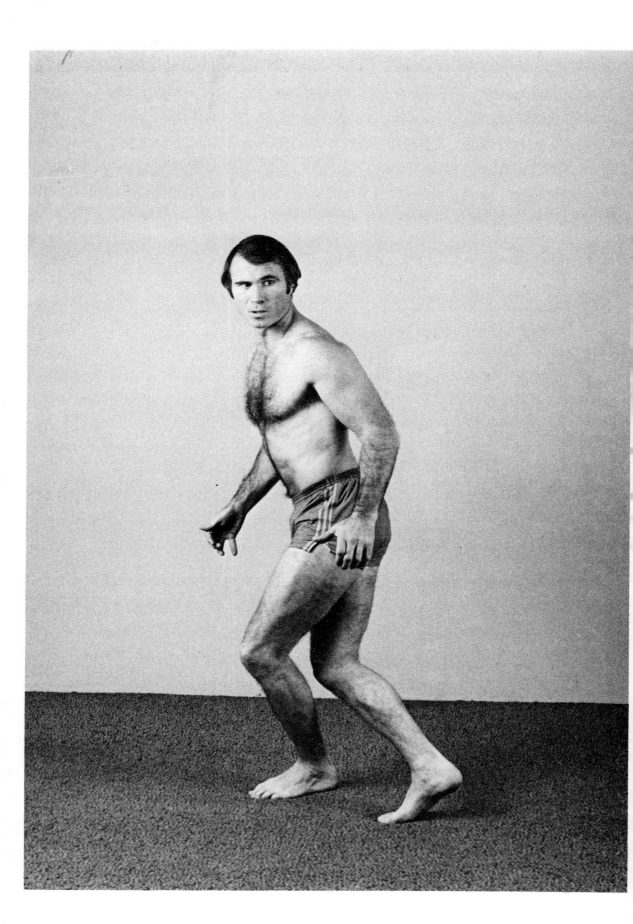

Footwork Exercises

Footwork exercises are total body exercises. To attain proficiency in these exercises, you need flexibility in all the major muscle groups. The legs must be strong and flexible; the upper torso must move smoothly; your balance must be superior. As you practice, you will discover where your weaknesses lie, and can concentrate on the exercises for those areas. Eventually you will bring together all of the improvements you have made through specific exercises to achieve total grace, agility, and strength.

Footwork Exercise #1

It's important to be able to vary your footwork when necessary, both to keep your opponent offguard, and to be able to follow your opponent when he changes his footwork. Each type of footwork pattern requires the development of different muscles.

Number of Repetitions

15-30 steps

Physiological Benefits

These exercises strengthen the calves, ankles, and thighs. They also enhance speed.

Martial Arts Benefits

Footwork exercises help improve your ability to close the gap and to move out of range of your opponent. By developing smoothness in these exercises you can avoid telegraphing your body positioning.

Pointers

Don't jump or bounce from step to step, but slide the feet evenly and smoothly. Try to keep your head level while your legs are moving. Keep the movement smooth and even. The body is relaxed and alert. Focus your eyes on an imaginary opponent.

Footwork Exercise #1

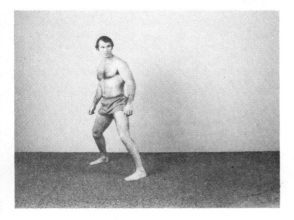

1. Stand erect with the feet shoulder width apart.

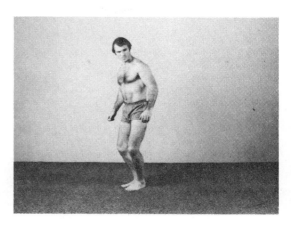

2. Slide your right leg up to your left leg.

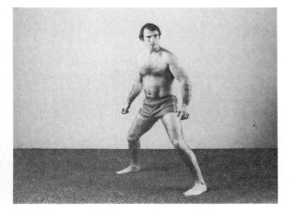

3. Slide your left leg out. Repeat this movement across the room.

Footwork Exercise #2

By practicing these crossing leg exercises you will get used to shifting your direction and position. Constant attention to variations in footwork patterns will increase your options in sparring: you will be able to move forward, cross over, or slide away easily.

Number of Repetitions

15-30

Physiological Benefits

In addition to strengthening the thighs, calves, and ankles, this exercise increases flexibility in the knee joint and improves coordination.

Martial Arts Benefits

The ability to shift directions and move freely in sparring can throw your opponent offguard.

Pointers

Don't try to move so quickly that you twist your knees. Strive to gain smoothness as well as speed. Do not be afraid to develop these exercises to fit your own special requirements. To adapt and enhance an exercise that you learn is also an important aspect of training and discipline. As you develop this particular exercise, experiment with it, execute the exercise at varying speeds and with varying distances in stride in all possible combinations. The movement will feel different when you are barefoot or wearing shoes. The type of terrain and ground you are on will also make a big difference. Being barefoot on a rug in your living room, for example, is completely different from wearing tennis shoes on asphalt. To keep the training and exercises interesting, you must develop a sense of imagination. This is a simple and practical method of self-motivation. Have you ever practiced footwork wearing leather-soled shoes on wet grass? Have you ever practiced footwork wearing hiking boots on the beach? If you have not, you will probably be in for a big surprise. Accept the exercise as a challenge and master it. If you can develop the ability to innovate, the simplest exercise can become the most advanced, the most outrageous exercise can become the most practical.

Footwork Exercise #2

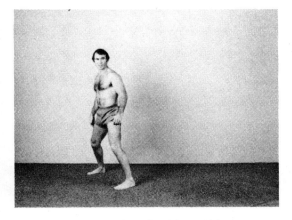

1. Stand erect with feet shoulder width apart.

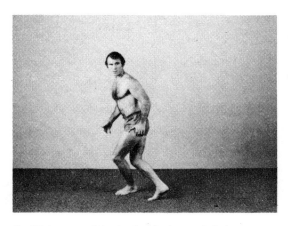

2. Slide your right leg behind your left leg.

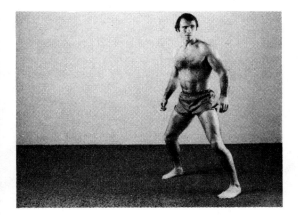

3. Step out with your left leg.

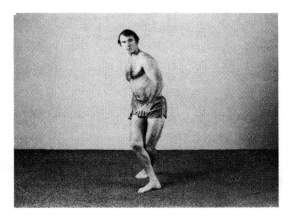

4. Slide your right leg in front of your left leg.

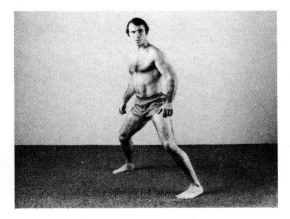

5. Step out with your left leg. Repeat in the opposite direction.

Footwork Exercise #3

The smoother you are in executing quick, intricate moves, the more easily you will be able to move smoothly and quickly in all phases of sparring.

Number of Repetitions
15-30 each direction

Physiological Benefits
The hip, ankle, and knee joints are lubricated and loosened. All the leg and waist muscles are toned.

Martial Arts Benefits
This exercise helps you develop mobility and smoothness, and to avoid telegraphing your moves.

Pointers
Don't overtwist your body in executing these moves, as this may put undue pressure on your knees. Try not to move your upper torso. Instead, rotate your hips more fully.

Footwork Exercise #3

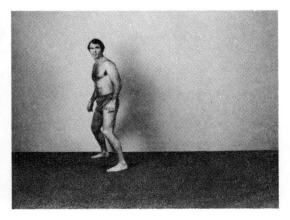

1. Stand erect, with feet double shoulder width apart.

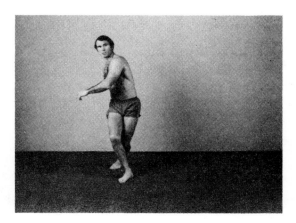

2. Bring your left foot behind your right foot. This time swivel your hips to the rear with each step.

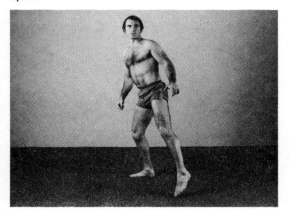

3. Step out with your left foot.

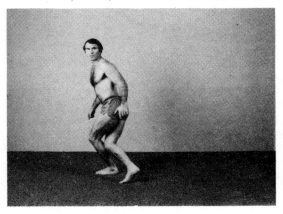

4. Bring your left leg over your right leg.

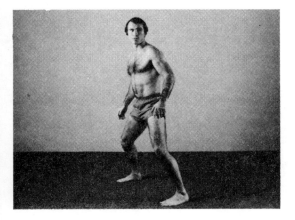

5. Return to the original position. Repeat in the opposite direction.

Footwork Exercise #4

Number of Repetitions
10-20
Physiological Benefits
This exercise strengthens and loosens the waist and ankles. It also improves your balance and body positioning.
Martial Arts Benefits
By improving your footwork you will be able to position your body for a kick smoothly, without telegraphing your movements to your opponent.
Pointers
It is essential to execute these moves very smoothly. Again, do not forget to focus on an imaginary opponent. This enhances your sense of balance, develops your sense of spacing between yourself and your opponent, and sharpens concentration.

Footwork Exercise #4

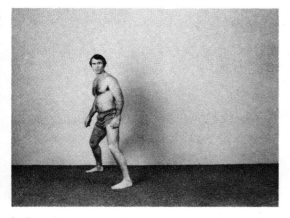

1. Stand erect, with feet double shoulder width apart.

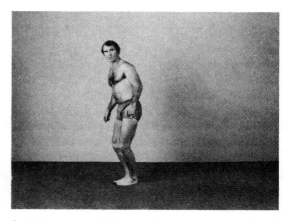

2. Slide your left foot up to replace the right foot.

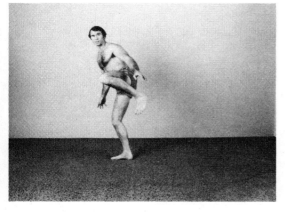

3. The left knee comes up as if being cocked for a kick.

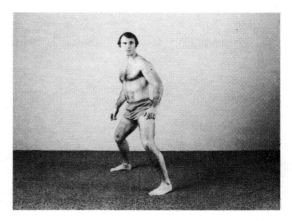

4. Then return to the original position. Continue the slide-cock movement.

KICKING

My Style of Kicking

I use three basic kicks in my style: the side kick, the roundhouse kick, and the hook kick. I use the same stance, footwork and knee position to deliver all three kicks. The opponent never knows which kick is coming until too late.

By adapting a side stance as opposed to a frontal stance, I am always in position to deliver my kicks without telegraphing my movement. Usually, there is a slight shifting and positioning of the hips before a kick is delivered; this warning gives the alert opponent the opportunity to block or counter the kick. My footwork is the same for all three kicks. I use a shifting movement of the feet which is quick and does not disturb the balance or position of my hips. My knee comes up in the same way for all three kicks. The knee protects my body and positions the leg to snap the kick out at the same time.

Because I have refined my movement to deliver all three kicks in exactly the same manner, my opponent must take the defensive; always wondering which kick he will be obliged to block and which kick will score the point. All three kicks can be executed in any combination. This skill, integrated with quick jabs and punches and the ability to close in and evade with speed, spontaneously produces an infinite number of techniques and combinations in mathematical progression.

Keeping my opponent psychologically on the defensive, I maintain control over the situation. This factor allows me to take the initiative at will. Initiative combined with the speed of the attack and the ability to flow into any other attack combination are the most important components in fighting and winning competition. This is the underlying principle of my style.

I don't want to tell anyone how they should fight or do their kicks. I don't expect the reader to accept everything written in this book or try to do it the way I show it. Take the little part that works for you and incorporate it into your style. Use what works; discard what doesn't. Don't sink to what is below you; rise above what is superior.

Developing a Style

I believe that it is important to develop your own personal style based on your strengths and weaknesses, limitations and potentials. This means that you must take a good, honest inventory of yourself both on a psychological as well as physical level. Refine your skills and use everything to advantage. I, personally, have an advantage in kicking and flexibility. This is what I constantly hone and sharpen.

In traditional karate training, your instructor says, "Do it because I say so." He really never tells you why. He usually teaches you the way he was taught. He thinks, "Whatever is good enough for me is good enough for you." This faulty logic is evident in all martial arts. We are each individuals and work within our own parameters. If you are to gain proficiency and mastery, you must have clear insight into yourself. By understanding yourself, you become innovative and creative. By becoming innovative for the sake of being different, you are simply falling into another trap that everyone else falls into.

You must create your own style. It is a way of expressing yourself. If you have three people from the same system do the same technique, none of them will look the same. For one, the technique may work very well. For the second, the technique may not work at all. For the third, the technique may be too easy or too difficult. Each individual has his own psychology, muscularity, speed, flexibility and strength. I don't believe in styles. Everyone has his own style.

My own style evolved out of my experiences in moving from point competition to full contact competition. In competition during the early sixties, the two fighters would bow in, and then take a hard fighting stance, toe to toe with each other. In those early days, the distancing was automatically set and there was hardly any jamming techniques at all.

Now everyone bounces around. The more sophisticated fighters know how to vary their positions and ranges. Judging distances is more difficult. Although this gives you time to set up your strategy; it also makes it easier to get your own techniques blocked or jammed.

My Stance

I do all three kicks from the side stance. There are several advantages to this.

1. You can deliver all three kicks from the same position, without telegraphing to your opponent which of the three kicks you are going to use. If you stand in the boxer's stance with your body and hands in a more frontal position, you will alert your opponent each time you shift your hips to kick.

2. You are less of a target in the side stance. In a frontal stance the groin and chest become ready targets for your opponent. In a side stance, the opponent has to angle around you to strike or punch.

3. You are in a better position to evade a blow in a side stance. In some cases, you can merely turn your shoulder to block a punch. Remember, if you have to block with your arms, you are leaving yourself open somewhere else. Never reach out to block.

4. You multiply your choices of action by utilizing the side stance. You can slide up in a straight line to kick. You can twist and punch to deliver a back fist. You can step back and punch. You can step back and kick.

Once you are in the side stance, it is easy to deliver all three kicks. You get into the position for kicking by sliding forward and pivoting simultaneously. Push off and then step. Practice it in three steps. The right leg replaces the lead leg. It is not a hop but a replacement. Your head stays level. Do not bounce. It is important to maintain a strong sense of balance in the base leg and hips. Eliminate all unnecessary body motion to avoid telegraphing your movement. This not only promotes smoothness but speed as well.

Front Stance and Side Stance

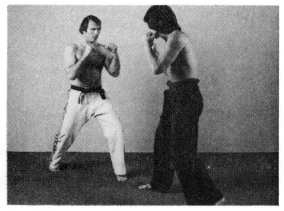

Front Stance.

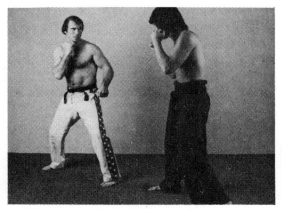

1 Side stance to basic kicking position.

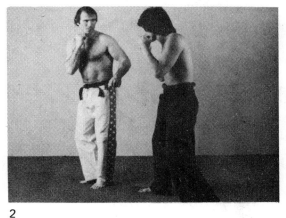

2

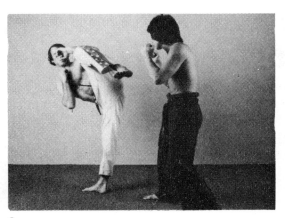

3

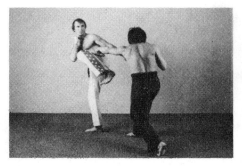

Incorrect position of knee from side stance to kick. Note: The knee is too low exposing the body to a counter punch.

Using My Kicks

White belts usually start out kicking a lot during sparring sessions. They get jammed and their techniques are consistently countered with a reverse punch or some other counter. When this starts happening too often, they give up kicking.

I've tried to find a way to get the kick out without leaving myself vulnerable to a counterattack. I want to be guaranteed that no matter what kicks I use, I won't be countered. Therefore, when I deliver my kicks, I use a speedy, snappy movement that gets the kick out and back quickly. If the kick hits its mark, that's fine. If it misses, that's fine also; it means my opponent is too far from my body to hit me. In addition, I keep my knee high to protect my body. I can actually hide behind my knee. I won't be countered because I protect myself throughout the entire movement. This is the secret of effective kicking.

For my kicking style, muscular legs are not essential. I, myself, have rather thin legs. For me, lighter legs move more quickly. I use abdominal muscle groups and quadricep muscles to lift my legs. If you do not develop abdominal strength, you can swing your leg, but you cannot develop speed and hold the leg up.

Snapping the Kick

I use a snap in my kicks instead of a thrust. Your power is transmitted through a very small part of the foot. When you snap the kick, all of your power is concentrated at that point. People used to say that snappy kicks have no power. They called them the "Wallace flippy-dippy kicks." These were the days before full contact competition. After the arrival of full contact competition, however, they saw—and felt—the actual power and speed of those kicks. Their attitudes changed considerably.

The snap is much easier on the knees than the thrust kick. A thrust hyperextends the knee joint as the weight of the leg pulls the joint outwards. Since I started snapping the kicks, I have not only increased the speed of delivery but eliminated many possible injuries.

By thrusting the leg out in delivering the kick, excessive pressure is exerted against the kneecap and joint. Over a period of time, the cartilage in the joint begins to break down. This condition is known as chondromalacia of the patella. The problem can become serious and usually accounts for the pain that most practitioners feel after working on their kicks. This wearing away of the cartilage is very similar to the irregular tread wear on the tires of cars not properly aligned. If you are developing these symptoms, change your technique immediately. This is why I use the snap in place of the conventional thrust.

Knee injuries have an indirect effect on your feet and hips. By favoring a bad knee or not taking proper care of an injury, you will throw off your footwork. Your hips will no longer move or shift smoothly. As a result of this, you will be telegraphing all of your moves to your opponent and the overall effectiveness of your technique will diminish greatly. This type of injury, as with all injuries, detract from your general health and well-being as well as your skill.

Snapping the kick is not only a safer method but a quicker method too. It allows you to get your kicks in and out of range effectively. You can take one position and launch a whole series of kicks in combination. Remember to keep your knee high for protection.

The Wallace Side Kick

The Wallace Side Kick is a snapping kick. When you snap the kick, its power is transmitted in a straight line. If your opponent tries to jam the kick, he will run right into it.

The traditional side kick uses two angles, instead of one straight line. By using two angles, you dissipate the effectiveness of the kick. The power comes at the instant the leg snaps out. If your opponent is too close or too far way, you lose power. Range is very important.

Use the side of the foot as the striking area for the side kick. Remember to start in a side stance position, and raise your knee high for protection. Do not slide up and then pivot your hips in two separate moves but slide and pivot the hips simultaneously. The movement is quicker and you telegraph less to your opponent. By combining all the elements of the kick into one movement, you increase your speed and eliminate excess and unnecessary motion. A direct movement is, in the case of the side kick, a more powerful movement. By increasing the speed and directness of the side kick, you reduce greatly the reaction time of your opponent, thus enhancing the overall effectiveness of the technique.

Side Kick

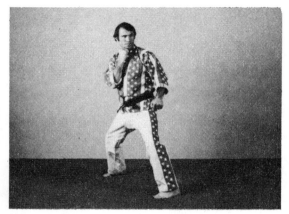

1. Side stance.

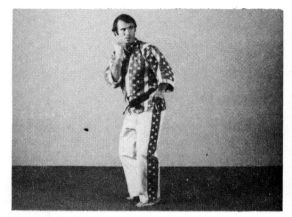

2. Slide the foot up.

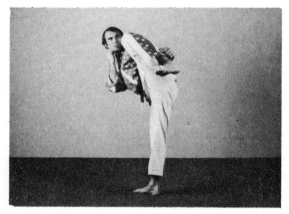

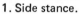

3. Cock the knee up.

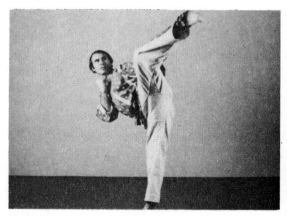

4. Snap the leg to target.

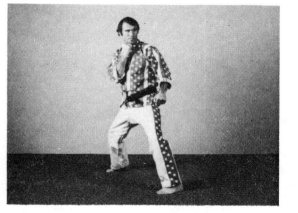

5. Return to original side stance.

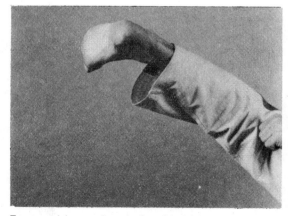

Foot position and angle for side kick.

Incorrect Side Kick

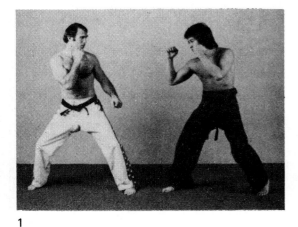

1

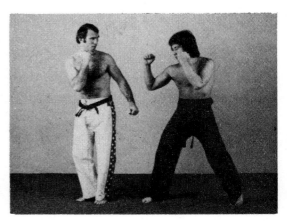

2

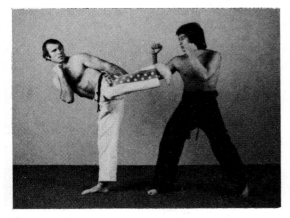

3

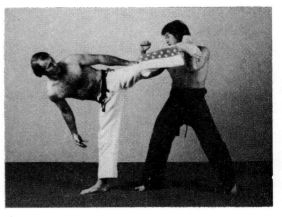

4

Incorrect side kick. The kick is thrust out not snapped. There is no elevation in the knee and the hips are turned away from the opponent.

The Wallace Roundhouse Kick

The traditional roundhouse kick is executed with the rear leg. It was always considered, until now, that only the rear leg could have any power. Traditionally, you kick with the ball of the foot.

Being left-handed and left-footed, I couldn't use the roundhouse kick with my rear leg without switching sides. I would always telegraph my roundhouse kick. It was necessary to adapt the roundhouse kick to meet my own requirements.

Now, I deliver the roundhouse kick from the same position as the side kick, using the forward leg. Although this is not the conventional method, I have found it to be quite effective. It also throws off and confuses my opponent. Sometimes, I can beat my opponent before he can adjust to my unconventional technique. The kick comes around rather than swings up and down. By making the movement gather force as it comes around, the kick becomes snappier and easier to work with in combinations. The delivery of the kick is also much quicker. Don't create an angle with this kick or you will leave yourself open to a counter.

Since my toes have never been able to bend back, I don't strike with the ball of the foot as the traditionalists do. My toes would always get mangled in the process when I tried to do it that way. I use the instep as the striking area. For myself, it is easier and more comfortable. This makes the technique more effective. Using the instep protects the foot. In addition, it extends the angle of the ankle and increases the hitting range by four to five inches.

When you execute the roundhouse, be sure you kick high enough. If the kick is too low, it can be blocked easily by your opponent. Keep your knee high for protection as always and kick from the side stance.

The effectiveness of this kick depends on the speed of execution and the power that comes from the balance in the support leg and the flexibility of the hips. Although my method may be highly unconventional, it may be, for some of you, a new weapon to add to your arsenal of skills.

Roundhouse Kick

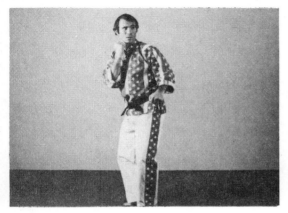

1. Slide up.

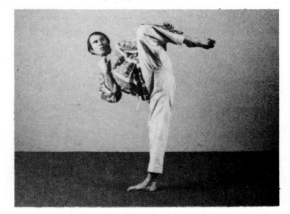

2. Cock the knee high.

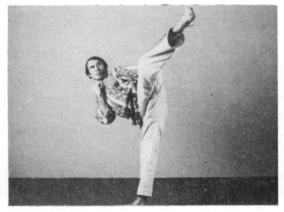

3. Snap out the leg.

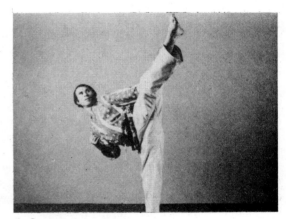

4. Completion of the snap.

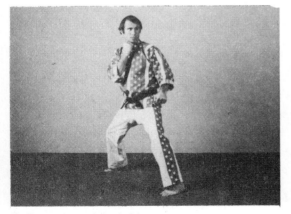

5. Return to original side stance.

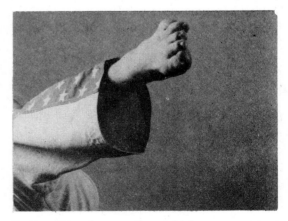

Foot position for roundhouse kick.

The Wallace Hook Kick

The traditional hook kick is executed by swinging an almost straight leg to the target area. This type of kick is easy to counter by stepping into it and jamming it. Once you jam the kick, your opponent is open and vulnerable to almost any attack or counter.

I throw the hook kick like my side kick. The only difference is at the end when I snap the heel through. My opponent does not know if I am doing a side kick or a hook kick until too late. It is very difficult for my opponent to jam or block the kick simply because he does not know which kick is coming. In executing the hook kick, it is important to keep the knee high. If the knee is lower than the foot, you are slapping your opponent, not kicking him. The effectiveness of the kick is greatly diminished. Also, you keep the knee high to protect your body during the kick. Always use the heel as the striking area for the hook kick. Only use the flat of the foot if you are in point competition.

By throwing the hook kick in this way, you increase your ability to work combinations on your opponent. After I snap the leg through with the hook kick, I can retract the leg immediately into a roundhouse kick position or I can turn the knee and follow through again with a side kick. There are many possibilities. I always keep the knee high in the same position. It is important not to lose your balance. If you lose your balance and step down, you will leave yourself open to your opponent's counter and you will not be able to work any combinations. Stay out of range.

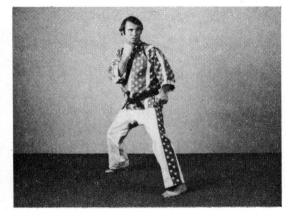

1. Side stance.

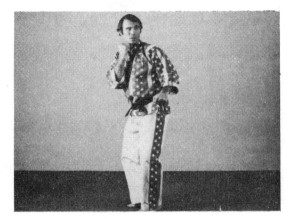

2. Slide up back leg.

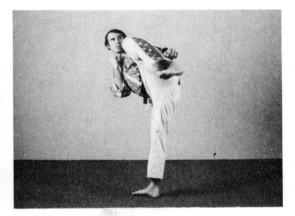

3. Cock knee up.

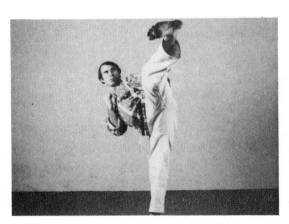

4. Leg hooks.

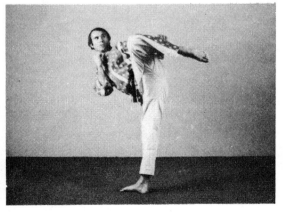

5. Leg retracts.

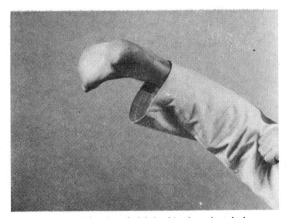

Foot position for hook kick. Notice that it is the same for the side kick.

Correct execution of hook kick.

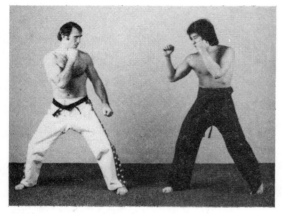

1. Assume stance.

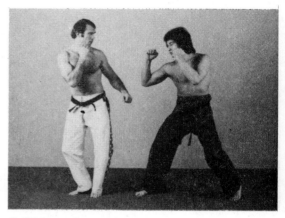

2. Slide up the rear leg.

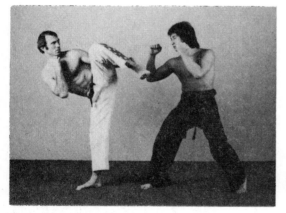

3. Cock the knee high.

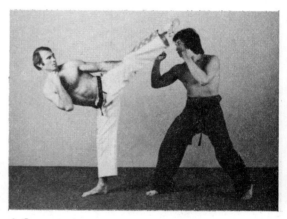

4. Snap the leg out.

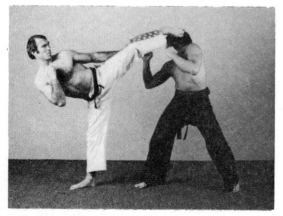

5. Hook to the target.

Incorrect hook kick. Notice that the knee is too low. If the opponent moves in, the body must turn away from the opponent losing balance and power.

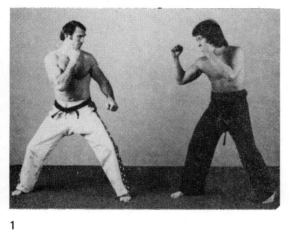

1

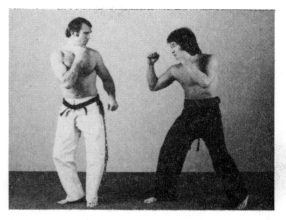

2

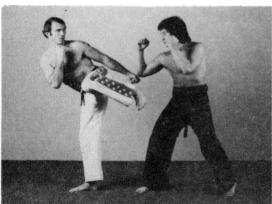

3

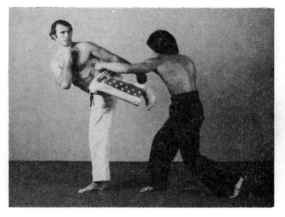

4

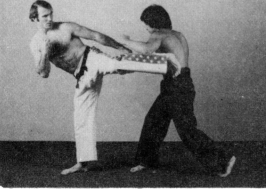

5

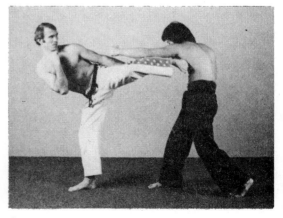

6

Analysis of Body Positions for Kicking

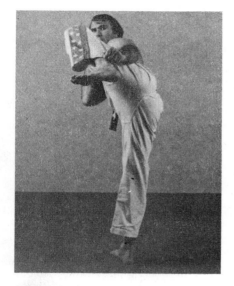

Correct body position. Notice the angle of the hips and the height of the knee.

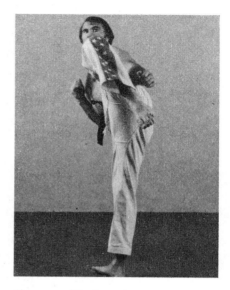

Incorrect. The knee is too forward and does not protect the body. The opponent can get around the knee.

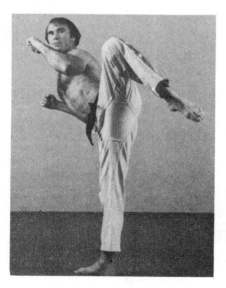

Incorrect. The angle of the knee is wrong. There is no stability and the groin and midsection is open to attack.

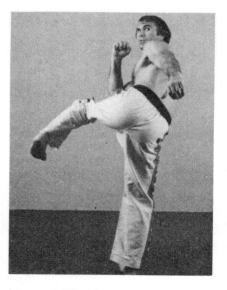

Incorrect. The hips are turned away from the opponent. There is no protection and the knee is not positioned for a direct kick.

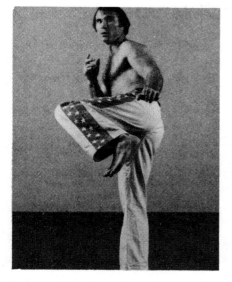

Incorrect. The knee is too low exposing the upper torso.

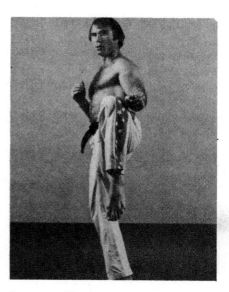

Incorrect. The knee is too low and the angle of the hips is wrong. The upper torso is exposed and there will be too much telegraphing of the kicks.

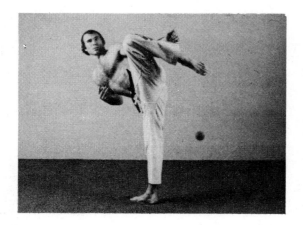

Correct knee position for kicks.

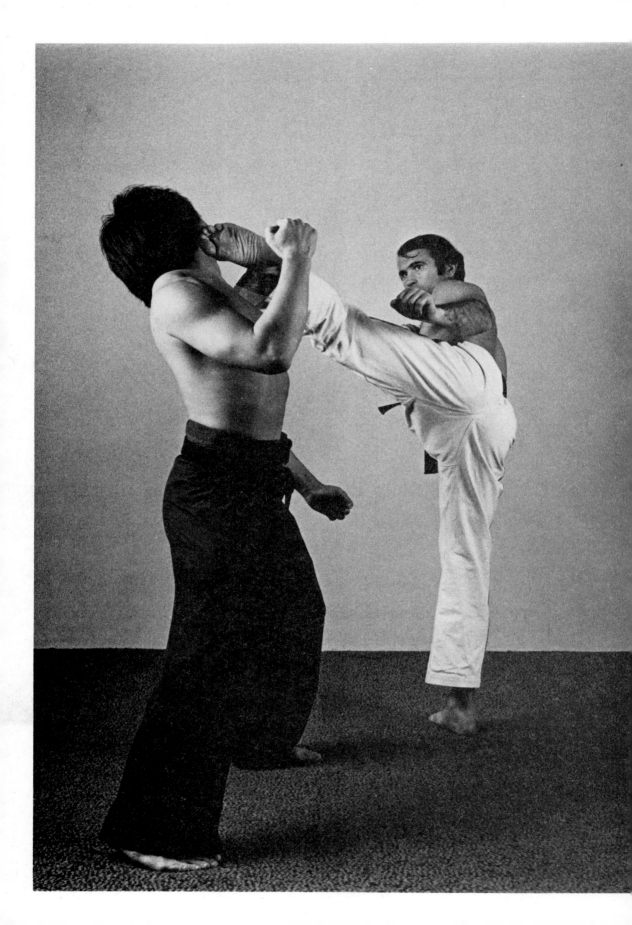

Combinations

Because I can use my three kicks in an infinite number of combinations, I can get through anyone's defenses to score. There is really an art to using combinations effectively. Fighting with combinations does not mean that you slide up to your opponent and just start throwing kicks at random. You must have complete mastery over each kick and develop the ability to deliver many kicks without losing your balance or stepping down. You must be able to evaluate your opponent's weaknesses and strengths very quickly and plan an effective strategy. You must learn how to immediately control the situation and take the advantage. In this way, you learn how to use your combinations to set your opponent up for the kick that scores.

Typical Combinations of Kicks

In fact, there are no set combinations of kicks, or any set order in which kicks should be used. Each individual has to develop his own pattern of kicking, which he bases both on his own and his opponent's strengths and weaknesses. Each individual has his own best technique. An instructor can teach the student how to execute the techniques correctly, but it's up to the student to discover what is most natural for him, and how to combine his best kick with other techniques in effective combinations.

My best technique is the roundhouse kick. It's easy and most natural for me. However, the roundhouse kick is also the weakest kick, because it's just a forward leg snap. For this reason, I know that if my last kick in a combination is a roundhouse kick, I have to be close enough to follow up with some other technique which will be more damaging.

Each student should evaluate his own best technique in this way. The roundhouse kick is a stunner, like a jab in boxing. The hook and side kicks are the power shots. As the student practices his kicks and tries to figure out the combinations that will work best for him, he should keep in mind that his easiest technique should be used to set up for his power shots. Joe Frazier, for example, would use every technique he had just to set up for his left hook.

Kicking Combination

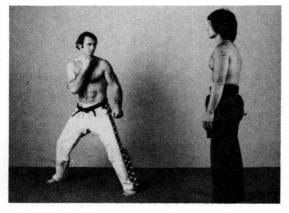

1. Assume side stance.

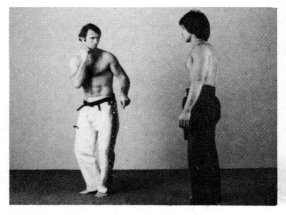

2. Slide up the rear leg.

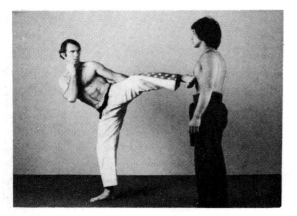

3. Side kick to the stomach.

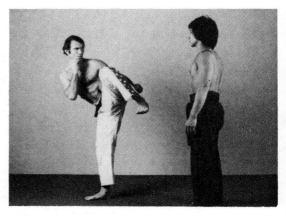

4. Snap the leg back.

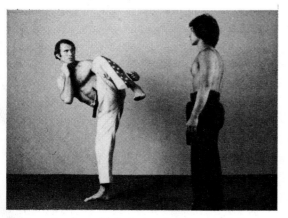

5. Keep the knee high and maintain your balance.

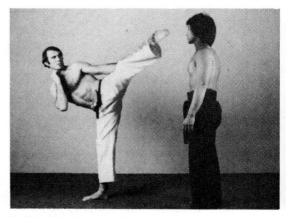

6. Hook kick to the face.

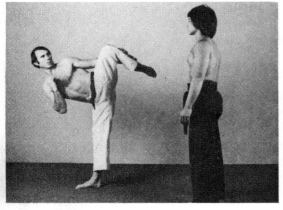

7. Snap the leg back.

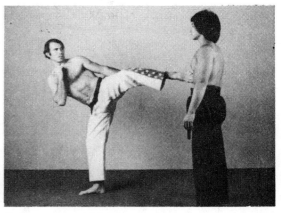

8. Roundhouse kick low to the stomach.

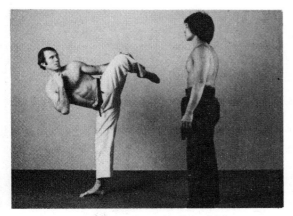

9. Snap the leg back. Keep the knee high.

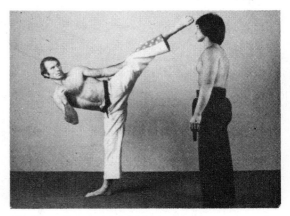

10. Roundhouse kick high to the face.

Side kick to stomach, hook kick to face, round-house kick low to stomach and completed by a roundhouse kick to the face again.

Practicing

To win with combinations requires strength, coordination, and balance. You must be very comfortable standing on one leg and delivering kick after kick. You must be able to quickly switch from kick to kick without changing your hip position or stepping down. Obvious shifts in the hips will telegraph your moves to your opponent. There are a number of training drills which will give you the skills for using combinations effectively in sparring.

The most important training technique is also the simplest: You should practice as many different combinations as possible. I practice with seven three-minute rounds of kicking combinations of three or more kicks. I try to come up with every possible combination or series of combinations. When I am working combinations, I am very relaxed, fluid, and rhythmic, like a dancer. I used to train to Simon and Garfunkel's "Bridge Over Troubled Water," which is about three minutes long.

Here are some sets of combinations to practice:

1. Double side kick. This is the hardest combination to master. The second side kick has a tendency to become a roundhouse kick. You have to be careful to bring the entire knee back, not just the foot.

2. Double roundhouse kick.

3. Hook kick, roundhouse kick at face level.

4. Low roundhouse kick, high roundhouse kick.

5. Side kick, hook kick, roundhouse kick high, roundhouse kick low, roundhouse kick high.

6. Low side kick, roundhouse kick, hook. Keep your knee in the same position.

7. Fake hook, roundhouse kick.

8. Fake roundhouse kick, hook kick.

Do not limit yourself to practicing just these combinations. Experiment with as many variations as possible.

It is important to learn to adapt your combinations to every possible situation of attack and counterattack. Be imaginative and innovative but always maintain a good, solid perspective on your training. If you are moving just to impress your opponent with fancy moves, you are missing the point completely. Be open to new ideas but test them out thoroughly in actual training and sparring. If an idea is not good or ineffective. Great! You can learn just as much from your errors as you can from your revelations. There is no easy road to skill and mastery. Therefore, it is of upmost importance to develop a positive attitude of constantly building on and refining what you know.

Partner training is an important aspect of building up your kicks. It is a good and effective method of developing your combinations, endurance and accuracy. Your partner should not be just a target or mannequin; he should provide you with constant motivation and feedback. He must be able to spur you on in your training and constantly remark on any and all weaknesses or faults in your movement. In this way, partner training becomes invaluable.

When practicing these combinations, sometimes execute the kicks very slowly, concentrating on keeping the knee in one position. Remember, you must learn to use all of your weapons from the same position. If your hips give away what technique you are going to use, your opponent will be able to counter you immediately. The only thing that should vary for each different kick is the position of your foot, and the area of the foot which you use to strike. I CANNOT STRESS HOW IMPORTANT THE POSITION OF THE KNEE IS IN MY PERSONAL STYLE. The knee protects my body while it maintains the position from which all my kicks are delivered. You need training and endurance to keep the knee high and also strengthen the support leg. Balance is also an important factor. By practicing slowly, you can better analyze the movement of the knee in relation to the kicks. If there is too much unnecessary movement in the knee, you will throw off the accuracy of your kicks and reduce your ability to keep your balance. At the same time, that unnecessary movement will alert your opponent to your kicks. Train to develop balance, smoothness and accuracy. These are the basic constituents for building up speed and strength.

Slide Up, Side Kick to the Stomach and a Roundhouse Kick to the Head

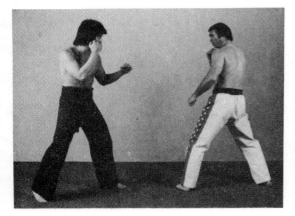

1. Assume stance.

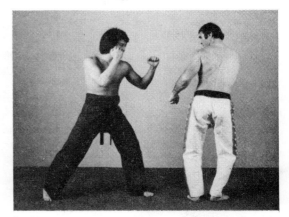

2. Slide up.

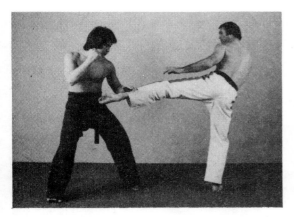

3. Execute the side kick low to the stomach.

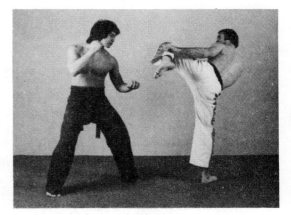

4. Cock the knee high.

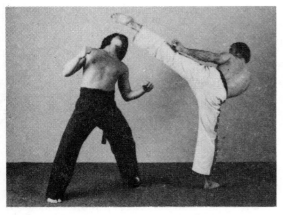

5. Execute roundhouse kick to the face.

Note: In the transition move to the roundhouse kick, be sure the knee comes high to protect the body.

Partner Training

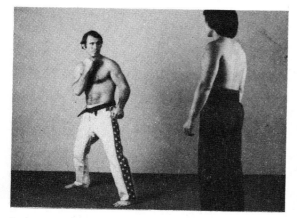

1. Assume side stance.

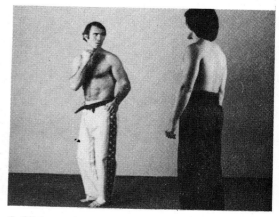

2. Slide up the rear leg.

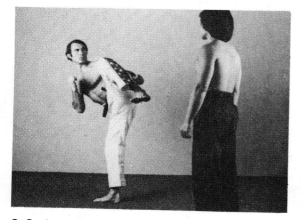

3. Cock the knee high.

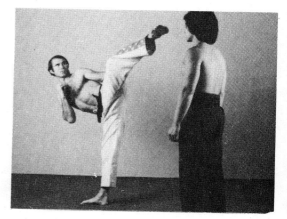

4. Execute side kick.

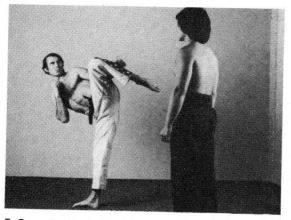

5. Snap the leg back.

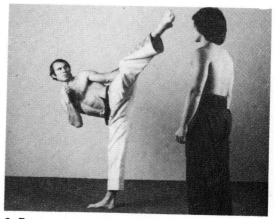

6. Execute roundhouse kick.

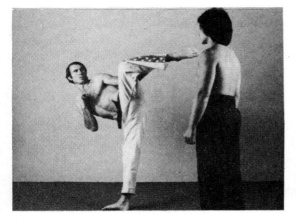

7. Follow through.

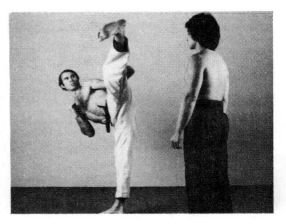

8. Execute hook kick.

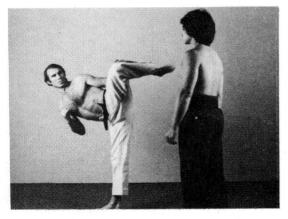

9. Follow through.

Practicing a combination of side kick, roundhouse kick and hook consecutively in one movement. Your partner provides you with an actual target.

Practice Exercises for Endurance

It is vital to have the stamina for delivering a series of quick kicks. By stressing repetitive practice of your combinations, you will be able to develop the muscles in your standing leg, your abdominal muscles, and the quadriceps. These are the muscles which help give you the endurance for a long, powerful series of kicks. The following are sample endurance exercises. However, you should be able to devise others.

1. Hold on to your partner. Roundhouse kick with your left leg, kicking the leg out and back ten times. Then switch legs and repeat. Do the same with the side kick and the hook kick. This improves reaction time and speed of movement, as well as endurance.

2. Spar with your partner for several minutes while both of you are standing on one leg only. Practice using different kicking techniques as you are hopping forward and backwards. Use your leg to jam, block, attack, defend, and counter, without putting your foot down on the floor. After you have been sparring in this way for two or three minutes, repeat with the other leg. Try extending each session to five or ten minutes. Eventually, when you are in an actual sparring situation, your opponent will only see your foot coming at him.

Practice Exercises for Targeting

No matter how good your kicks are, you will not be able to score unless you are able to place them exactly where you want them. It's no good throwing a roundhouse kick to the stomach and hitting an elbow. You should practice foot-eye coordination constantly. Eventually, you will be able to use your foot like a hand.

1. Pick a target and practice hitting it with your foot. You must train to be able to hit the target not 99 times out of 100 but 100 times out of 100.

2. Practice working a speed bag with your different kicks.

3. When you're sitting at home watching television, reach for the television dial and touch it with your foot.

Targeting ability must be developed along with balance, coordination, and strength.

Endurance Training With a Partner

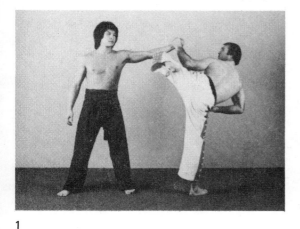

1

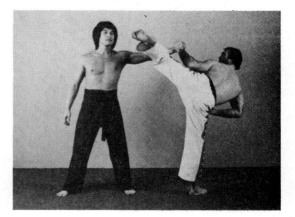

2

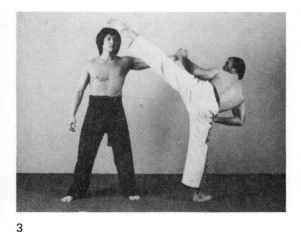

3

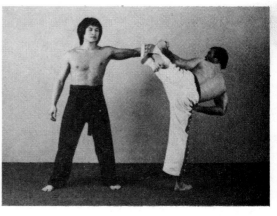

4

You use your partner to stabilize yourself as you practice your kicks. The important point is to develop stability in the hips and keep the knee high. Your partner is an invaluable aid to your training but should never become a crutch. (Note: You can prevent this by always increasing the difficulty of the exercises and creating new challenges for yourself.)

Endurance and Accuracy Training

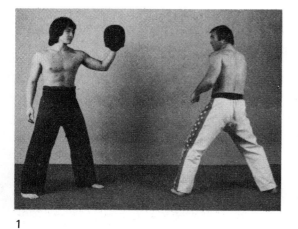

1

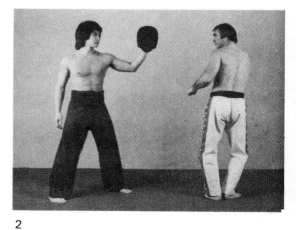

2

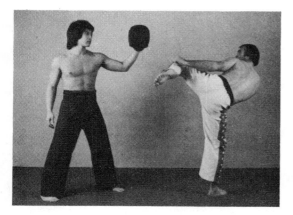

3

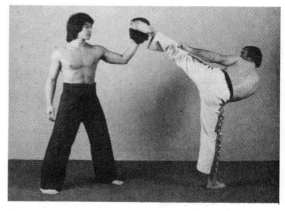

4

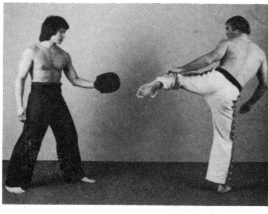

5

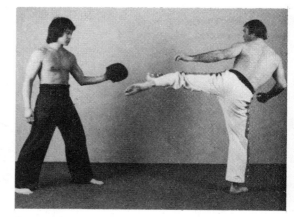

6

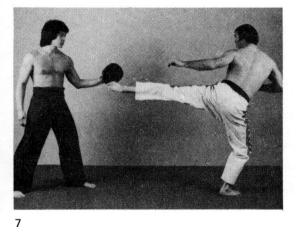

7

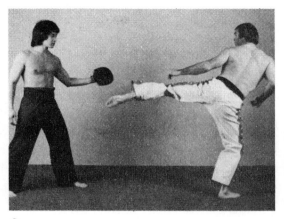

8

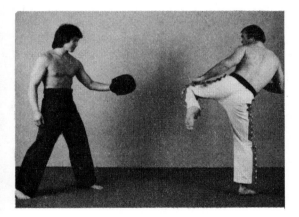

9

Practice a combination of kicks as your partner randomly moves the mit. Be able to target in on the mit ten times out of ten. Notice how well the body is balanced on the support leg and how the knee of the kicking leg is kept high for protection at all times. Note: If you must step down between kicks, your balance is off or your support leg is too weak. By stepping down, you lose your combination, break your timing and open yourself up. This is very dangerous.

Clearing: The First Kick

It's no good trying to use combinations if you never get your first kick out. If you have a combination in mind to use against your opponent, use your first kick as a clearing device. It is vital to clear the way first. For example, you may have a roundhouse kick-hook kick combination in mind. You start your roundhouse kick. But what if your opponent is a jammer? As soon as he sees you move, he'll move towards you, and you'll never get the hook out.

I use the side kick as my clearing kick. The power in a side kick comes out in a straight line. This means the kick won't be jammed. After clearing the way with a side kick, then you can shoot out your second kick. The second kick is used to set your opponent up. The third kick is used to score. Remember, you don't want to strike your opponent with the clearing kick. If I hit you with the side kick, you will be knocked back. You won't be there for the second kick.

The Second Kick: Setting Up Your Opponent

After clearing the way with a side kick, you want to use another kick to set your opponent up for the scoring kick. If you don't set a kick up before you throw it, it'll probably just hit a block.

In boxing, you're standing close enough to your opponent so that all your punches can hit. It's different in sparring. Once I'm on one leg, the opponent can do something which I can't: He can move. When I'm up on one leg kicking, I have to be sure of what the opponent is doing and what I'm doing. To be sure of your opponent, you have to test him to see how he reacts.

Don't throw hundreds of kick combinations immediately. First, for 15 to 20 seconds, throw kicks only to get your opponent's reactions. Don't worry about getting the kicks in. Right now you just want to see how your opponent moves. How does he react to hand techniques, single kicks, your stepping? Does he jam, back up, put up his hands to protect himself?

Throw the first hook kick as fast as possible. Your opponent may back up, come forward, drop his head, or raise his hands. I don't care, since I'm standing far enough back that I know the opponent can't get to me. Just snap that kick in and out. Then try another kick. After you spot his typical reaction pattern, start targeting your kicks. This is similar to your tactics in the first round in a boxing match, when you're just feeling your opponent out.

Keep your opponent from jamming by keeping your knee high. Then come over or around his block, or step down and use your hands or leg to stop his technique. The leg is like a buffer zone.

What kicks you finally decide to throw depends on how your opponent is reacting.

1. If your opponent tries to jam, try throwing a short hook kick to his face and simultaneously drag the rear leg six to seven inches forward. Then you're in range to roundhouse kick to the face without stepping again.

2. If your opponent starts blocking with his hands, you're in great shape, because he can't block everything. In this situation, I start working combinations; when your opponent blocks, he's open somewhere else. No matter how fast he is, it takes time to block. I can just fake a kick, and he'll bring his elbow down to block it.

3. If the opponent moves back, none of the combinations will work. In this case, you have to catch your opponent off guard, when his weight is on the forward leg. I try to work an explosion, a quick snappy motion towards the opponent to surprise him. I take one quick, explosive step to get me close enough to the opponent to start working combinations. Some fighters spin to cover the distance, but I don't believe it's necessary. I only need that one step to get very close.

The kicks to set up the opponent are used not only to see how your opponent reacts, but also to condition your opponent to react the way you want him to. People used to say about me, "He's throwing kicks just to be throwing kicks." But actually, I was throwing kicks to have the opponent lower his guard so I

Clearing and Setting Up Your Opponent

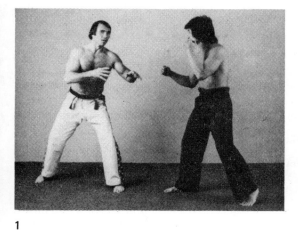

1

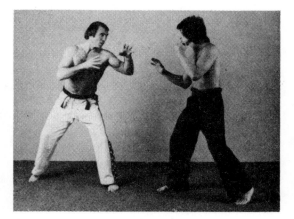

2

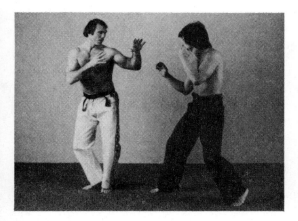

3

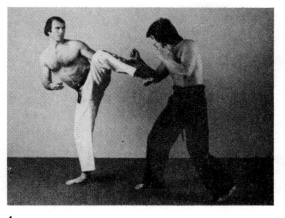

4

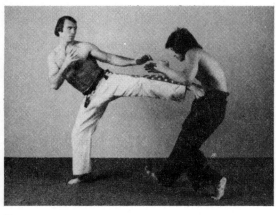

5

Side kick to stomach. The side kick is effective for clearing the way for your combinations. If contact is made, your opponent will not be there any more.

could get through and score. Here are a few examples of how to train your opponent to react in predictable ways:

1. Try throwing a low roundhouse kick three or four times at the opponent. As you keep throwing the low roundhouse kick, your opponent's hand will automatically start dropping. Then you can get him with a high roundhouse kick.

2. You can keep throwing hook kicks at your opponent until his head automatically moves away. Then get him with a low roundhouse.

Faking to Set Up Your Opponent

By faking a kick, you can set your opponent up for your scoring kick. My favorite is to fake a hook, then throw a roundhouse. If the opponent ducks every time I fake a hook, he's putting his head down in just the right place for a roundhouse kick.

I use faking when my opponent has taken a very hard stance, just waiting for me to move. I also use it when the opponent is really moving around and I can't get a bead on him. I fake something to see how he'll react.

Here are some examples of faking a kick to set up for the scoring kick:

1. Use a fake hook to set up for a roundhouse kick. The opponent acts the same way whether you're faking or throwing a real kick—he'll lean back. I throw the first three or four hook kicks very quickly, so he can't jam them. When I see that he leans back, I fake another hook kick, raising my leg half way straight. The opponent thinks a hook is coming, and leans back again. Then I fold the hook kick into a roundhouse kick.

2. The reverse strategy to the above can also be used. I fake a roundhouse kick and deliver a hook kick. When the opponent leans away from a roundhouse kick, he puts himself in the perfect position for a hook.

I fake the roundhouse enough times so I know the opponent's reaction. This usually takes two or three fake kicks. Then I slide up for a roundhouse kick, and begin folding my leg. The opponent leans back. Instantaneously, I fold the kick underneath, and deliver a hook kick.

Distractions

The art of distraction is a very important skill to develop. You distract your opponent to create openings, to make time, and to exert a psychological control over the situation. This skill is important in fighting as well as competition.

Just put your hand or leg somewhere your opponent will see it momentarily and take notice of it. The moment he uses to shift his attention to the hand or leg is the same moment you use to initiate your attack. Distraction and faking work together on the same principles and basically result in the same effect.

If I strike my arm out, the opponent will naturally react. He thinks it might be a back fist or a grab. He freezes momentarily, tensing his muscles, focusing his attention, trying to figure out and react to a movement that really has no meaning at all. You use his distraction to your advantage. Any movement can be a distraction. The important point is to catch the opponent's attention and draw it away from the real moves. Your real intention is completely different from what you are leading your opponent to think or believe.

A distraction will have no meaning whatsoever to the opponent if the movement does not appear "real" or carry "weight." In much the same way a mime might produce the effect of weight or movement while performing on the stage, you must have body language to distract the opponent. A mime might appear and give the impression of holding a glass of water and drinking from it when, in reality, he is not. It is an effect. You may appear to lead with a right jab when, in fact, you are not. You have another intention; you are setting him up for a roundhouse kick to the head.

Faking a Low Roundhouse Followed by a High Roundhouse

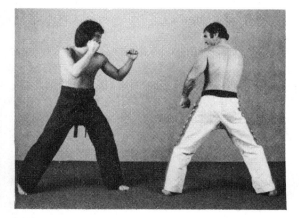

1. Assume stance.

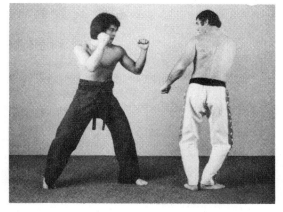

2. Attacker moves in to punch.

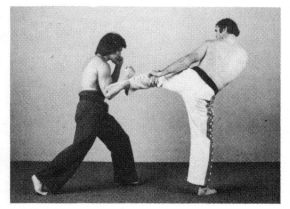

3. Faking low roundhouse kick.

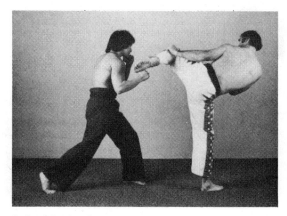

4. Positioning knee.

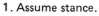

5. High roundhouse to face.

Note: I cause a reaction by faking a low kick to bring the opponent's guard down low and then I come in with a high roundhouse kick to the face. The low kick creates the opening and the high kick is the target.

Executing a High Kick and Followed by a High Roundhouse Kick

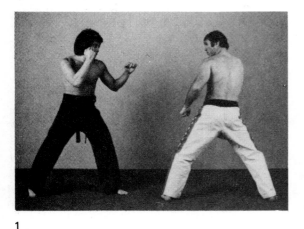

1

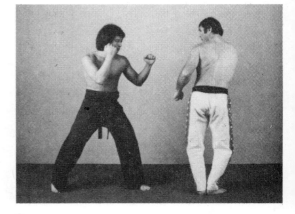

2

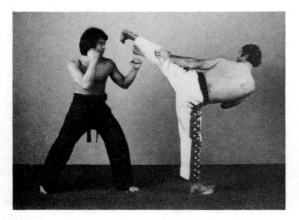

3

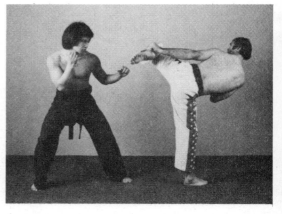

4

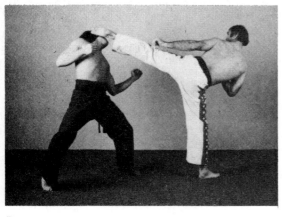

5

In this instance, a high kick does not cause the opponent to react. However, anticipating a low kick to follow, he drops his guard opening himself up to a high roundhouse.

The effectiveness of combinations relies heavily on how well you know how your opponent will react. Combinations are not governed by rules or forms. Combinations are created by circumstances and necessities.

Faking a Hook Kick Followed by a Roundhouse Kick

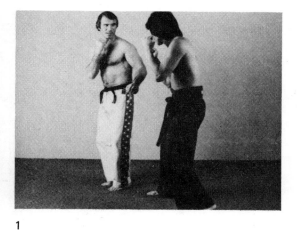

1

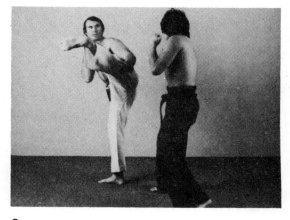

2

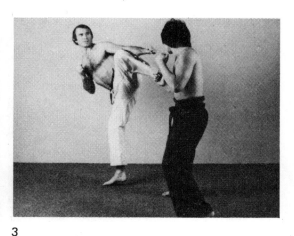

3

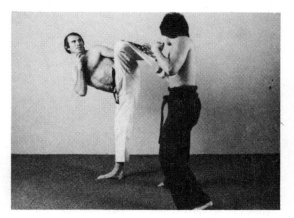

4

Raise the knee high and snap through with a hook kick causing your opponent to move away. Follow immediately with a roundhouse kick in the same motion. Note: The fake is used to determine your opponent's reactions and create openings for your techniques.

Faking With a Roundhouse Followed by a Hook Kick

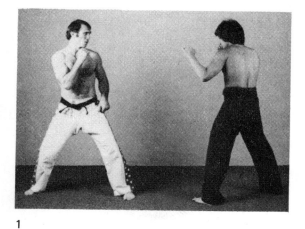

1

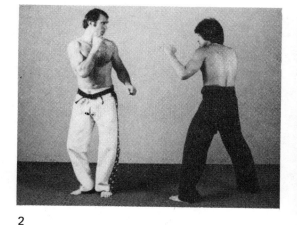

2

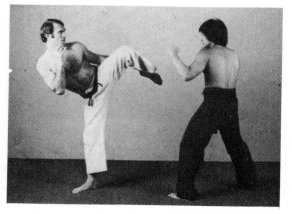

3

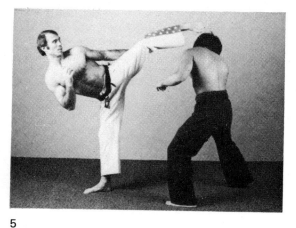

4

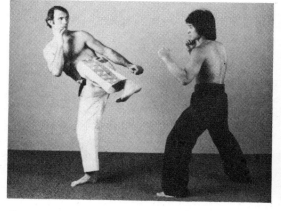

5

In this instance, the combination is reversed. Use a roundhouse kick to create a distraction and opening and follow with a hook kick to score.

Hand Techniques:
Using the Hands to Set Up Kicks

Hand techniques can be used to set up a scoring kick, much as fakes and kick combinations are used. I usually use a back fist, jab, or left hook for this purpose.

When throwing hand techniques, you should stand in the same side stance you use for kicking. You shouldn't have to change your stance whether you strike or kick. Any changes in movement telegraph your intended technique to your opponent.

When I'm testing my opponent's reaction, I'll throw some back fists from four to five feet away. I'll watch to see if he brings his forward hand up to block, or if he leans back, away from the strike. Ninety-nine out of 100 times, he won't try to jam a back fist. The back fist is too quick a movement, and it comes out straight, making it difficult to jam.

If your opponent brings up his hand to block the back fist, he is opening his body for a side kick. When you see that the opponent reacts consistently in this manner, a side kick is your next move.

If your opponent leans back, he is opening his body for a hook kick or roundhouse kick.

If your opponent keeps his hands in front of him, you will be able to use a hook kick. You can't use your roundhouse kick in this situation.

If the opponent begins turning, you can use a counter spinning back kick. I don't use this sort of maneuver; I prefer to back up and start again.

All of the hand techniques are basically used in the same way. They elicit a reaction from the opponent. Then you react to his reaction.

Hand Combinations to Hook Kick

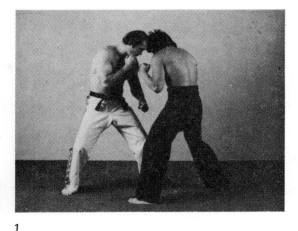

1

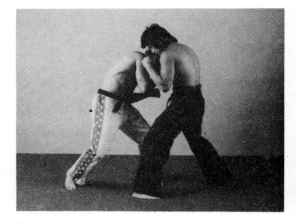

2

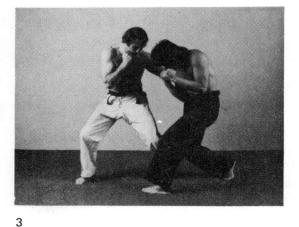

3

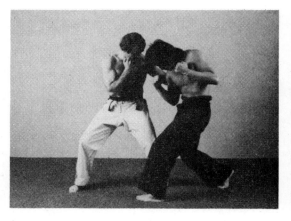

4

In this instance of in-fighting, a left hook is used to open up the opponent and position the body sideways. As the body turns, the knee is cocked and a hook kick is executed. Note: In any in-fighting or close range situation, where kicking combinations are not effective, use the hands to open up your opponent and create enough distance for the scoring kick.

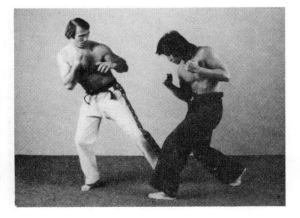

5

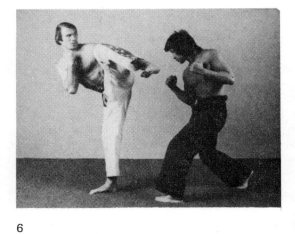

6

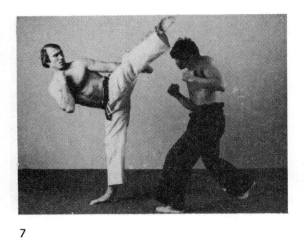

7

8

Back Fist Followed by a Hook Kick

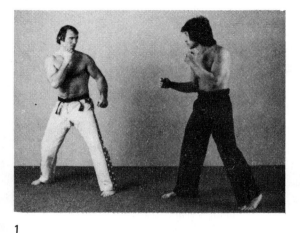

1

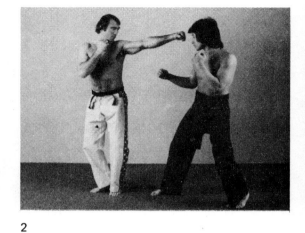

2

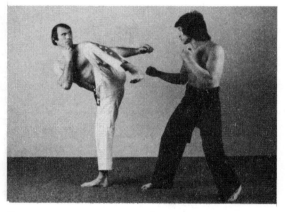

3

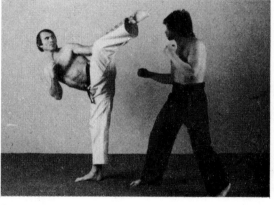

4

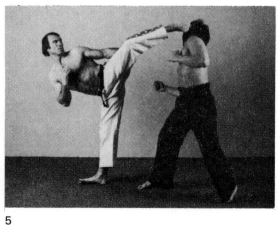

5

By sliding up and executing a back fist to the face, you can many times cause your opponent to move back. As he fades back, catch him with a hook kick.

Back Fist Followed by a Side Kick

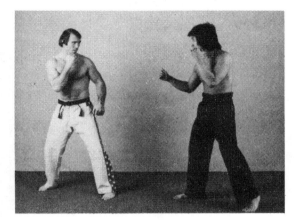

1

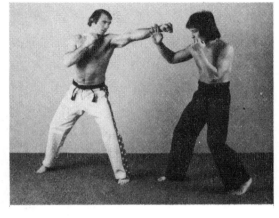

2

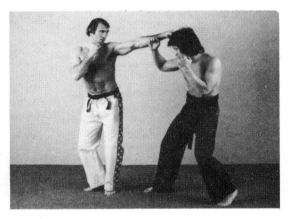

3

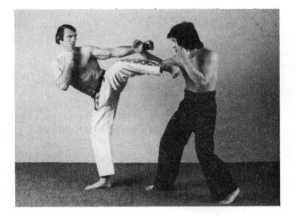

4

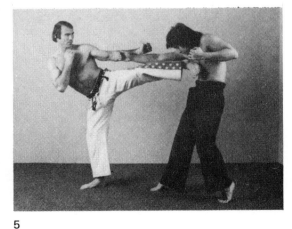

5

Execute a high back fist to cause your opponent to react by raising his guard. Slide up to close the gap and catch him with a side kick to the mid-section.

Distancing

My philosophy regarding distancing is quite simple: I won't take the chance of getting hit. I don't want the opponent to be able to reach out and touch me without taking a step. He shouldn't be able to hit me without moving. If your opponent is in range, he will be able to hit you, because the hand is quicker than the eye. But if he has to step first, you can react the minute he steps.

You can do almost anything to get out of your opponent's range. I get out of his distance by kicking, backing up, or moving sideways. If I'm not sure of what my opponent is doing, I simply back up.

I am only in range when I'm doing work. Then I get in quickly and out quickly. If I'm close enough to hit him, then he's close enough to hit me. I don't want to depend on blocking, because every block opens you somewhere else.

As long as you allow adequate distance, you will have time to react. Speed isn't as important as distance.

Distancing for Side Kick

Incorrect distancing.

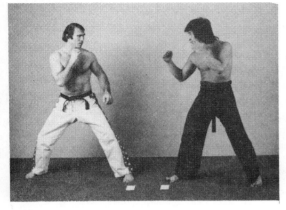

1. From the side stance.

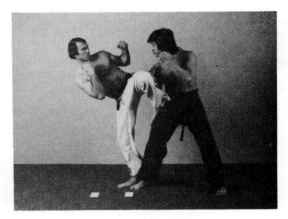

2. Opponent is too close jamming the kick.

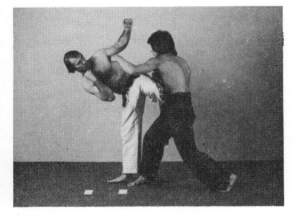

3. Opponent counters with a punch.

This is an example of incorrect distancing by sliding in too close on your opponent before the kick. The kick is jammed and the body is exposed to a counter.

Proper Distancing for the Side Kick

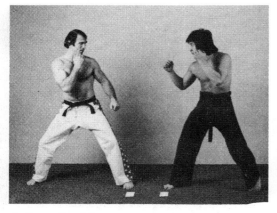

1. From the side stance.

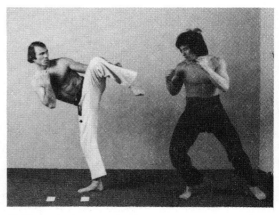

2. Opponent moves back.

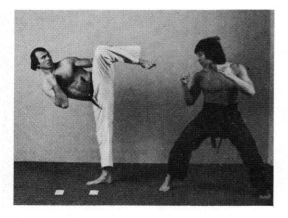

3. Knee is cocked high.

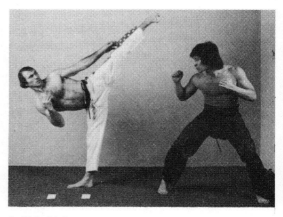

4. Side kick.

Incorrect Footwork Effecting Distancing

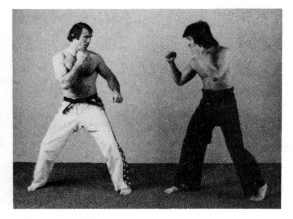

1. From the side stance.

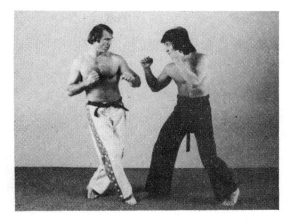

2. Incorrectly crossing the legs in front.

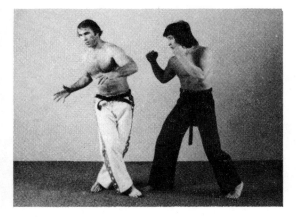

3. One's own kick is jammed and the body is exposed.

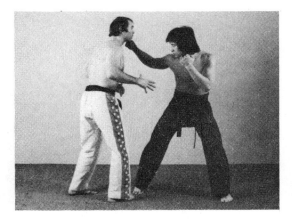

4. Opponent counters with punch.

Incorrect Footwork Effecting Distancing

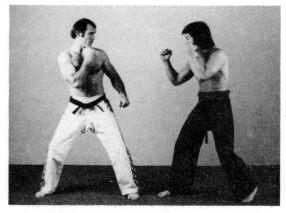

1. From the side stance.

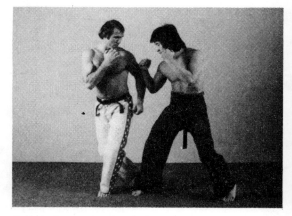

2. Rear leg crosses behind.

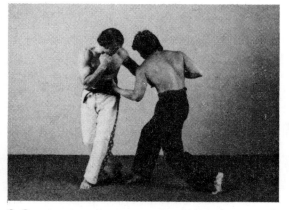

3. Opponent counters to exposed body.

If you cross your feet behind, you open yourself up to his punch and your kick is jammed.

Distancing with Feet Together (Sliding up from side stance)

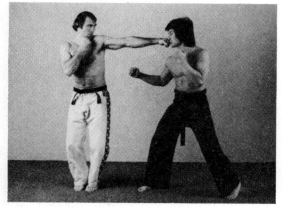

You can jab with the feet still together.

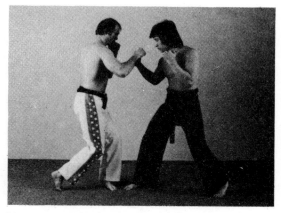

You can step back, pivot and follow through with a straight right fist to the face.

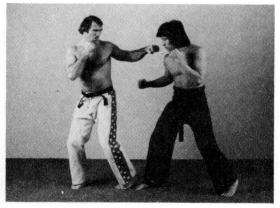

You can execute a left hook.

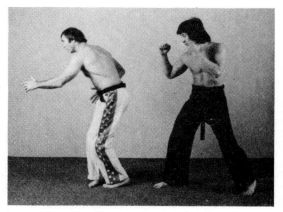

In a critical situation, you can turn tail and run the other way.

You are at a distinct disadvantage when you cross your legs in front or behind when moving in towards your opponent. I always use the slide up movement of the feet from the side stance. This allows me to execute any kick and maintain the proper body angle which does not expose me to a counter. This also allows me many alternatives I can punch or jab, execute any kick, continue to adjust my distancing or body angle or turn tail and run if I have to in a real situation.

Single Kicks

I use single kicks, rather than a combination, when my opponent is slow, or if I already have set up my opponent with a series of kicks or strikes.

There are a number of situations in which single kicks are appropriate. If both the opponent's hands are up, I can kick him in the stomach with a roundhouse kick. If the opponent's hands are covering his stomach, I can get his face area.

If the opponent uses spins, you need a different strategy. If his left side is forward, I might use a roundhouse kick to the body. If his right side is forward, I use the hook kick or side kick. I wouldn't use a roundhouse kick to the body or a left hook to the head in this case.

If I'm in close, and I see an opening, I may throw a single kick in order to create an opening for another single kick. You can see that there is a fine line between single kicks and multiple kicks or combinations. You need to be adaptable, constantly reacting to your opponent's reactions. After you work a single kick, see what your opponent does. He may be giving you an opening for another kick.

It may not be a disadvantage to have only one kick. For example, anyone who fought Joe Lewis knew he only had the side kick. But when you fight with him, you always wonder when that kick is coming. If you back fist him, you know his side kick is on its way.

For the last 15 years I've only thrown three kicks, and I only use my left leg. But my opponent doesn't know when it's coming or from where it's coming from. And just knowing it's coming works against the opponent—he's always on his guard, always a little stiffer.

Defensive Kicks

A defensive kick is a kick you use to react to your opponent's technique. You don't want to block when different kicks are thrown at you. If you block, it means you're too close to your opponent. By keeping your distance, you can see where to counter. If he throws a punch, he's open to a kick to the body. If he throws a kick to your face, his face is open, as he must lean back for balance. Here are three things to keep in mind when you are on the defensive:

1. Keep your distance. When in doubt, back up.

2. Know where your opponent is throwing his technique, and what technique he's using.

3. Instantly be ready with a counter for his technique.

I always want my opponent to throw something at me. This gives me an opening to use my techniques. Here are some examples of reacting defensively to an opponent's techniques.

1. My opponent throws his right hand. I lean back, and throw a defensive hook kick to his face.

2. The opponent throws a jab or back fist. I lean back, and throw a defensive side kick to his lower body.

3. The opponent throws a roundhouse kick from the rear leg. This puts his right side forward. I stick out a side kick and let him run into it. As he steps down, I throw a hook kick. This kick will always get in, because as the opponent steps down he relaxes his guard for a split second.

4. The opponent slides up for a roundhouse kick. I counter with my roundhouse kick without taking a step, because my opponent has already bridged the gap. While he's stepping, his legs are busy. My legs will be free.

5. The opponent throws a side kick. If I'm close, I'll bring my knee up to protect myself and to jam. Then I stick a side kick into the opponent's stomach or ribs.

6. My opponent throws a ridge hand. He's close enough so he thinks he can hit me. I lean back, throw a hook over his guard to the back or side of his head.

7. My opponent throws a jab. I bring a side kick up, and throw it under his guard.

8. My opponent is a multiple kicker. I must be able to instantly counter his counter, using the same kick.

Evading Punch Followed by a Defensive Roundhouse Kick

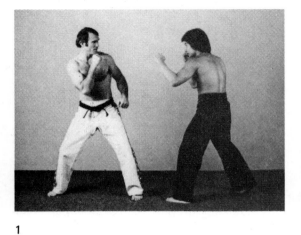

1

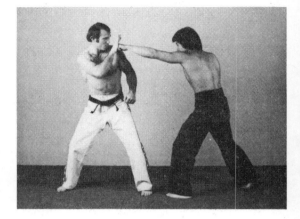

2

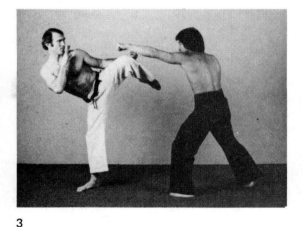

3

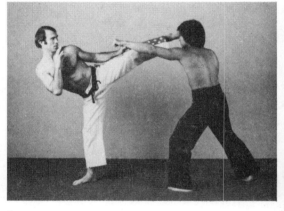

4

This is an example of evasion followed by a defensive roundhouse kick. The best defense
is to fade back away from the opponent's attack giving yourself enough distance to execute your kick.

Evading Punch Followed by a Defensive Hook Kick

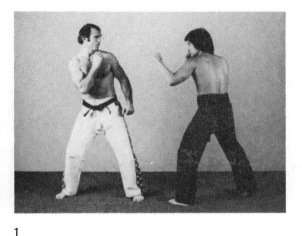

1

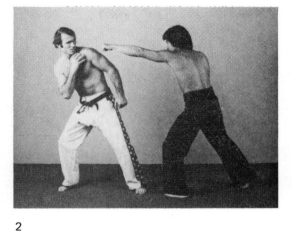

2

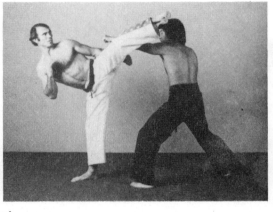

3

4

This is another example of utilizing a defensive hook kick. Speed is important to catch the opponent as he is still moving in with his attack. Do not give him a chance to recover his position or counter.

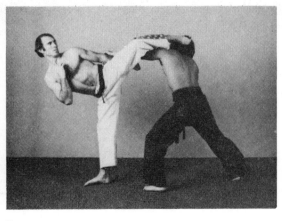

5

Evading Punch Followed by a Defensive Side Kick

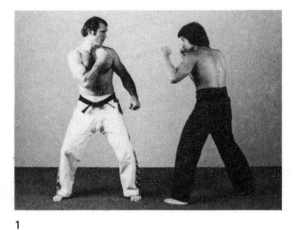

1

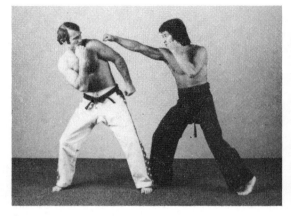

2

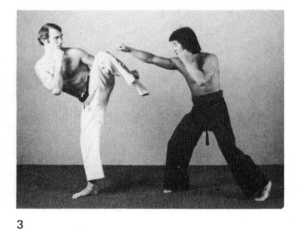

3

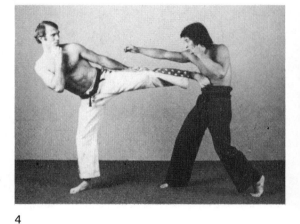

4

Evade the blow by moving back and counter with a side kick. When in doubt, step back. By blocking the blow, know that you are too close to your opponent and opening yourself up to his counter.

Defensive Hook Kick in an Infighting Situation

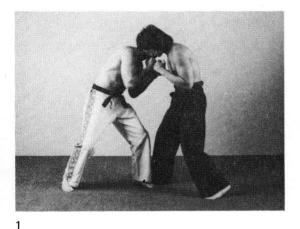

1

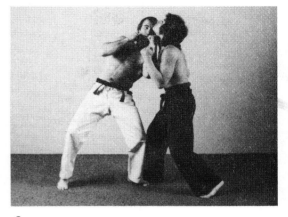

2

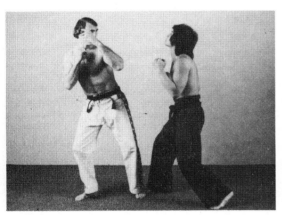

3

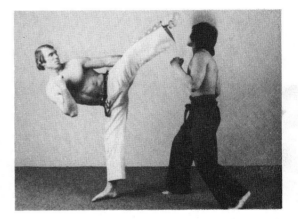

4

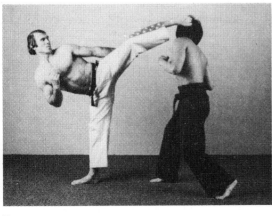

5

In an in-fighting situation, it is still possible to evade and counter with a defensive kick. In this instance a left hook kick to the side of the head is utilized. Note how foot position is important to achieve the proper distancing for the kick.

Jamming

Jamming is one of the most important techniques in the repertoire of a full contact fighter. Jamming has a number of unpleasant effects on your opponent. By jamming his techniques before he gets them started, you disturb your opponent's thinking and his balance. You keep him from making a big movement towards you, since he always has to be guessing whether you'll jam him or back up. If you're too close when he starts his technique, it will be stopped before it has any effect. If you're too far away, he'll throw his technique into the empty air and look like a fool.

Here are a number of pointers for jamming an opponent's technique:

1. Move almost simultaneously with your opponent. Short circuit his movement. You should be able to stop the opponent's technique before he can execute it.

2. Have an idea of whether the opponent is throwing a hand or foot technique. You will be able to tell by his stepping movement or his body movement. Watch the extremities, and see if a hand or foot moves. If your opponent lunges, he will probably be using a hand technique. If his hip moves, or he steps, he will be using a foot technique.

3. If you have determined that your opponent will kick, use your forward leg to jam. As soon as the opponent starts his forward movement, bring your knee up and to the side. Come forward and jam the person's forward movement before you do any other technique.

4. Always have in mind what you're going to counter with after you jam your opponent's technique. Don't jam and then stop, with no other move planned. Stop his technique by jamming the area, not the technique, and simultaneously counter the attack.

Counter Techniques to the Jam

1. Jam a side kick and counter with a back fist.

2. Jam a roundhouse kick and counter with a roundhouse kick or hook kick.

3. Jam a reverse punch with the arm close to the body and counter with a defensive hook or a back kick. It's easy to jam a reverse punch because your opponent has to step forward and turn.

4. Jam a side kick by leaning, and letting the kick slide over your shoulder. Then counter with a defensive hook kick.

5. Jam with your forward leg, and then counter with a strike to the body or head.

Jamming a Kick with the Knee Followed by a Roundhouse Kick

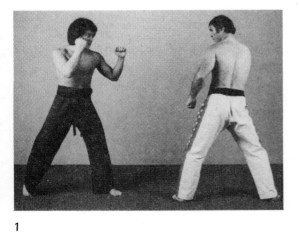

1

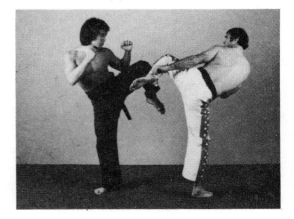

2

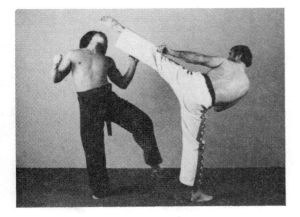

3

Jam the opponent's kick and follow through with a defensive roundhouse kick. In addition to evasion, jamming is another important method destroying the opponent's attack and countering with a kick. Jamming has the added advantage of also breaking your opponent's balance.

Jamming a Kick with the Knee Followed by a Hook Kick

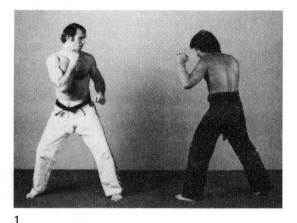

1

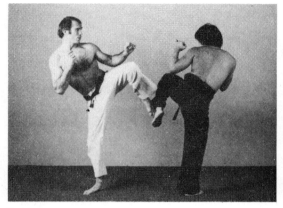

2

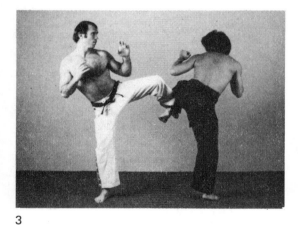

3

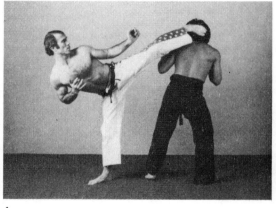

4

This is an example of jamming followed by a hook kick to the side of the head. The jam increases the opponent's recovery time restricting his counter to your kick.

Jamming a Punch with the Knee Followed by a Hook Kick

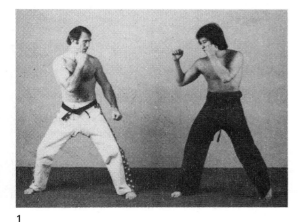

1

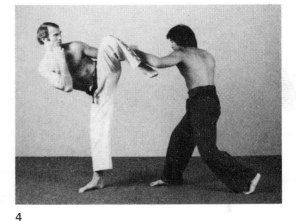

2

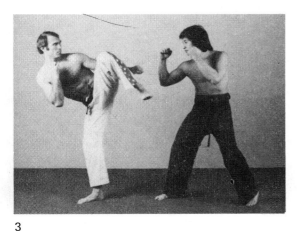

3

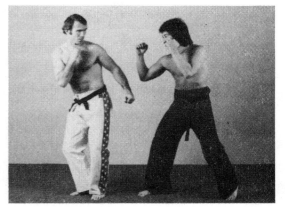

4

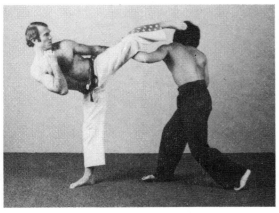

5

Using the high position of the knee to block the punch the jam is followed through with a hook kick to the head. Note that the knee position for the jam is the same as for the kick. From the jam you just follow through in a single movement. By avoiding all unnecessary movement, the technique becomes exceptionally fast and effective.

Evasion and Jamming Combined with a Hook Kick

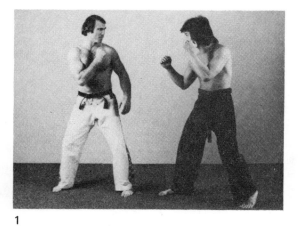

1

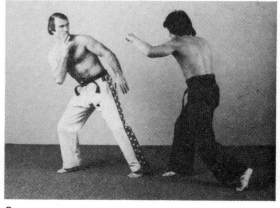

2

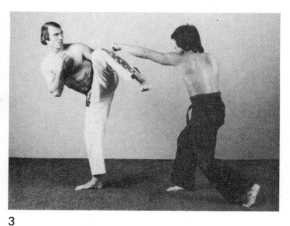

3

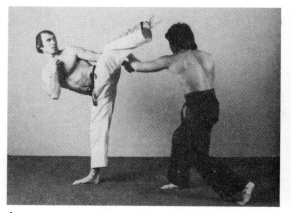

4

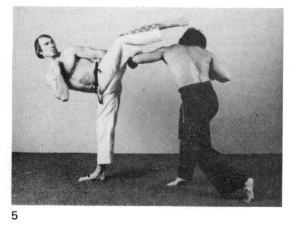

5

This example combines a slight evasive movement and knee jam followed by a defensive hook kick to the head. Note that in sparring, the basic movements and strategies evolve into an infinite number of patterns and variations.

In Summary

There is an old maxim in martial arts, "Train for a lifetime, and you will fall short of the mark; be lazy and negligent for one day, and you have already lost the match." Be patient and persevere and you will develop yourself without fail. All the exercises in this book from the very basic to the very advanced have all been helpful to me in my own training. I am passing these training methods on to you but please keep in mind that the main ingredient for success does not come from this book but from your own effort, sincerity and will.

I would like to end this book with another maxim from the martial arts, "Pure gold does not fear the test of fire." Be honest in your training and you will always, without fail, realize your aspirations.

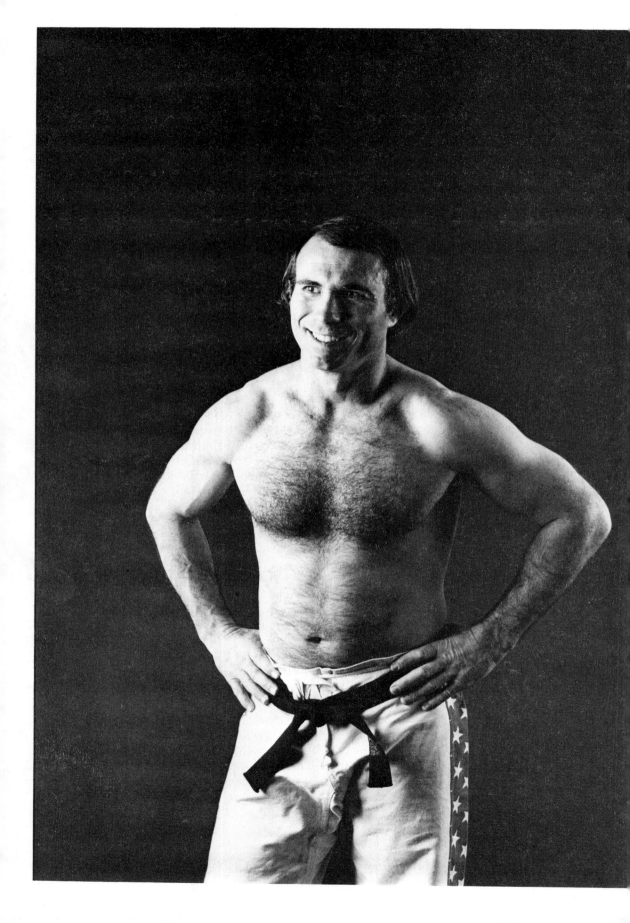

About the Author

Bill Wallace retired as the undefeated PKA middleweight karate champion after defeating Bob Biggs by a decision in the 12th round in June 1980. Ending Wallace's fifteen year career in karate, this bout also marked his twentieth consecutive victory (with 11KOs) in full contact competition.

Known as Superfoot for his celebrated left leg, which has been clocked at a delivery speed of 60 miles per hour, Wallace prides himself on using his foot as another fighter might use his hands, hitting opponents with two or three kicks in rapid succession, reaching under, over, and around their blocks, and placing kicks with amazing precision.

Even before entering full contact in 1974, Wallace was rated three times by *Black Belt* magazine as the top fighter in the country, and had won virtually every major tournament title. Among his successes were winning the U.S. Championships three times, the USKA Grand Nationals three times, and the Top Ten Nationals twice.

In 1973 Wallace sustained a leg injury, and it seemed likely that he would be unable to continue his competitive career. However, Elvis Presley, whom at the time he was instructing in karate, flew in a Los Angeles acupuncturist to treat the champion at Graceland Manor. Wallace permanently recovered his kicking ability from that treatment, and in 1974 in Los Angeles he became the PKA middleweight champ by defeating Bernd Grothe by knockout in the second round.

Wallace lives in Memphis with his wife, Susie, and two children. For several years he taught karate, judo, wrestling, and weight lifting at Memphis State University, the institution from which he earned a masters degree. He has authored a college textbook on karate and kinesiology.

Now Wallace also has a burgeoning movie career. He starred in *A Force of One* with Chuck Norris, and is currently slated to appear in *Neighbors,* with John Belushi, for whom Wallace has acted as body-guard and personal karate instructor. Wallace plans, however, to return eventually to his teaching position at Memphis State.

In a recent interview in *KICK Illustrated,* Wallace insisted that he has left the karate ring for good. Only one thing would change his mind. "The only reason I would come back is if the sport starts getting sloppy. If that happens, then I'll come back and try to clean it up."

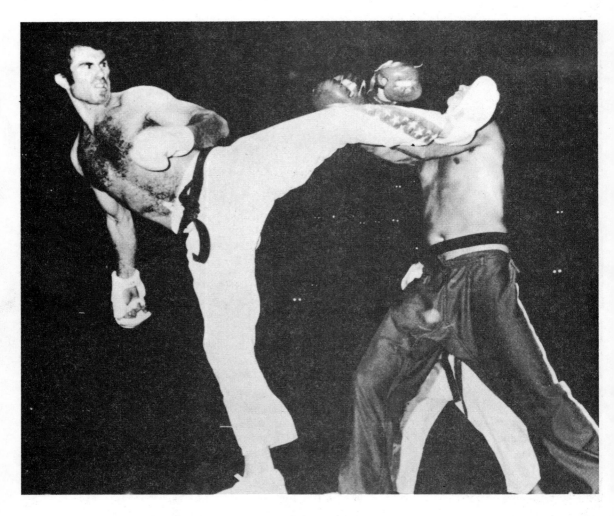

Above: 1974, Los Angeles: Knocking out Germany's Bernd Grothe to win his world middleweight full-contact crown.

Opposite Top: The Champion making his screen debut in 1979 in 'A Force of One' with Chuck Norris and Jennifer O'Neill.

Opposite Bottom: Another scene from the same movie.

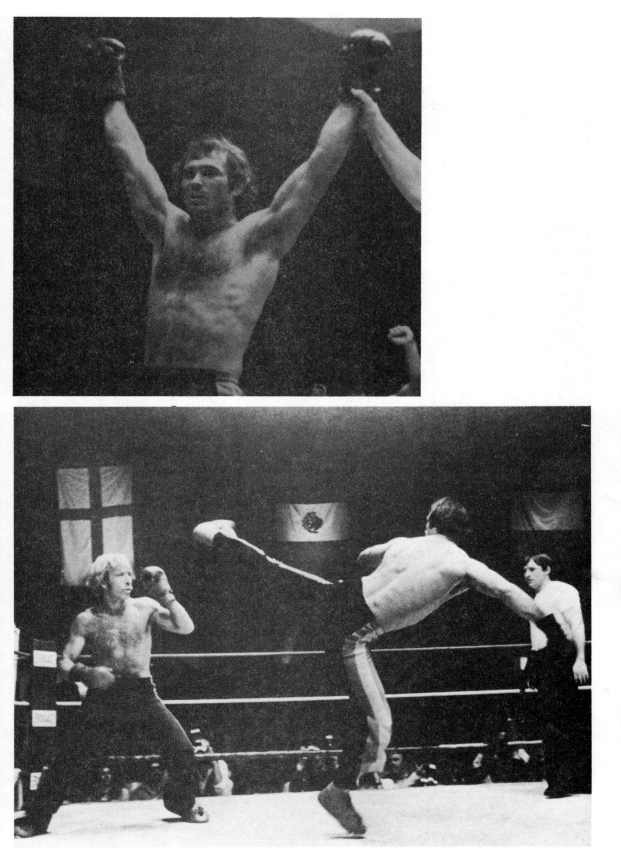

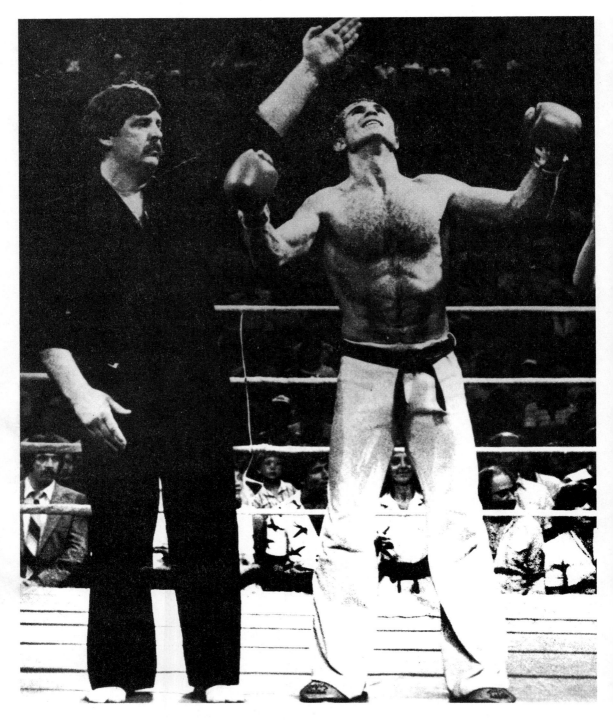

The Champion, Bill 'Superfoot' Wallace.